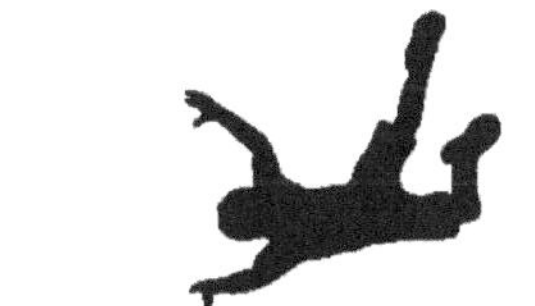

GREATER

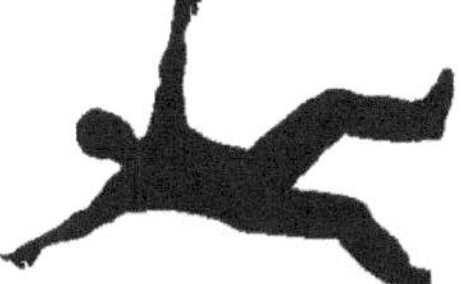

THAN

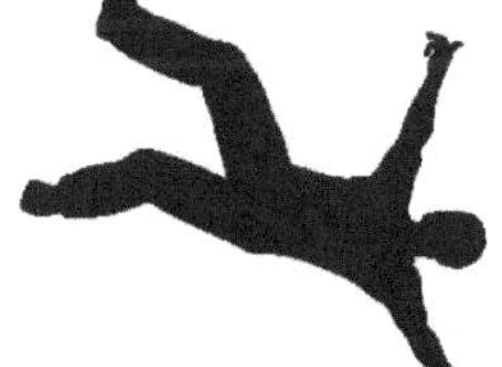

GRAVITY

ISBNs

Paperback: 978-1-968559-01-4

Hardcover: 978-1-968559-00-7

ebook: 978-1-968559-02-1

Published by UACT Press

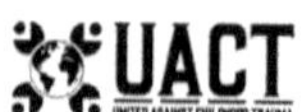

Praise for Greater Than Gravity

"Truly a beacon of hope, illuminating the path to wholeness and self-empowerment."

As a therapist treating adults, I'm constantly seeking deeper understanding of trauma and healing pathways. Menard delivers exactly that—and more.

Childhood trauma casts a long shadow on an individual's life, and this book illuminates every corner of that shadow with remarkable clarity. The detailed explanations and logical progression make complex trauma concepts accessible to any reader, regardless of background knowledge.

What sets this work apart is its perfect balance: comprehensive information presented through digestible methods that empower rather than overwhelm. Readers gain both understanding and actionable tools to combat this epidemic.

I cannot recommend *Greater Than Gravity* strongly enough—it's genuinely eye-opening and transformative.

Mary J. Dowd MA, LCAS, LCMHC, CCSEMDR
Therapist & Clinical Supervisor, Treehouse Recovery
Intensive Outpatient Program

"Hope remains, and this book is its voice."

In the ancient Greek myth, Zeus, ruler of the gods, was determined to punish humankind by sending Pandora to live among them with a sealed jar. Curious, she opened the seal, unwittingly releasing epidemics of sickness and famine and war.

Since the turn of the 21st century, healthcare researchers and clinicians have understood that sickness and violence and substance abuse and even early death have a common root, and that root is childhood trauma. The original study that documented this truth has been replicated numerous times across a variety of cultures and countries. Yet somehow, policymakers and even many clinicians, have remained unknowing and thus powerless.

In Pandora's jar, one thing remained: hope. Michael Menard's work is that hope. In *Greater Than Gravity*, he explains both the neurological and the societal impact of childhood trauma in ways both personal and accessibly academic, then offers a blueprint for a way forward. This is not only a book to be read—it is a book to be enacted for the sake of our children and our grandchildren.

Hugh Marr, Ph.D., clinical psychologist
Author of *A Clinician's Guide to Foundational Story Psychotherapy: Co-changing Narratives, Co-changing Lives*; and of *Finding Your Story: Using Archetypes to Guide Your Personal Journey*; co-author (with Carol Pearson, Ph.D.) of the Pearson-Marr Archetype Indicator

"This book will inspire action and foster the change our world so desperately needs."

In writing this (sadly) very necessary and important book, *Greater Than Gravity*, Michael Menard has demonstrated true bravery and dedication.

With passion and purpose, he masterfully weaves lived experiences, personal stories, science, and a wealth of research to reveal the urgent need to address childhood trauma—not only for individuals, but for our communities and society as a whole.

What touched me most is the clear emphasis on prevention and hope, especially the clarity given to the essential need for secure attachment in the earliest days of life.

Greater Than Gravity is sure to make a significant contribution to the growing movement toward healing and prevention.

Deborah McNelis, M.Ed.
Author of *The First 60 Days*, Founder, Brain Insights and
creator of Neuro-Nurturing

"Menard's gift as a master storyteller brings humanity to the stark statistics."

Michael Menard is extraordinarily qualified to be a spokesperson for the movement to eradicate the silent epidemic of Adverse Childhood Experiences (ACEs). A survivor of multiple ACEs himself who rose from a 900-square-foot home below the poverty line to become a world-renowned innovator with fourteen patents, Menard brings both lived experience and exceptional brilliance to this crisis.

In *Greater Than Gravity*, he eloquently explains how childhood trauma wounds the mind, body, and spirit, while offering fresh and powerful solutions. As only a passionate person who has "been there" can, Menard's gift as a master storyteller brings humanity to the stark statistics—transforming cold data into a compelling narrative that will inform, inspire, and help those who have survived childhood trauma, those who care about affected loved ones, and those who desire to prevent this enormous suffering.

Childhood trauma and its disastrous repercussions in adulthood is a colossal global epidemic, costing the American economy alone trillions of dollars annually.

Despite research consistently confirming the link between childhood trauma and everything from depression and addiction to cancer and heart disease, this epidemic remains largely unrecognized. Menard has devoted himself to making sense of these complexities and turning useful ideas into practical solutions that can be applied on a large scale.

This remarkable book represents hope and healing for millions affected by childhood trauma.

Glenn R. Schiraldi, Ph.D., LTC US Army (ret.)
Stress Management Faculties at the Pentagon, University
of Maryland, and the International Critical Incident
Stress Foundation
Author of *The Adverse Childhood Experiences Recovery
Workbook, The Post-Traumatic Stress Disorder Sourcebook,
The Resilience Workbook,* and *The Self-Esteem Workbook*

In memory of Patrick and Adam.
In honor of every child who deserves better.

All of the stories in this book are true. In some circumstances, names and identifying details of several individuals have been changed to protect confidentiality. Some vignettes are retold from the author's previous published works.

The content of this book is based solely on my personal experiences and the insights gained from conversations with individuals and literature produced by experts in the field, including but not limited to Dr. Glenn Schiraldi, Dr. Nadine Burke Harris, and Dr. Bessel van der Kolk, as well as those listed in the acknowledgment section of this book. I do not possess any formal education or training in medicine, psychology, or therapy.

This book contains material that may be emotionally challenging for some readers; if you find yourself struggling with the content, please prioritize your well-being and feel free to pause or discontinue reading at any time.

In *Greater Than Gravity*, I share my journey and perspectives regarding childhood trauma, its impacts, and potential pathways to healing. It is not to be interpreted as professional advice, medical diagnoses, or trauma treatment. I encourage readers to seek qualified professionals for guidance regarding their own experiences and mental and physical health.

Contents

Foreword

Greater than Gravity is an eye-opening book about the human suffering caused by toxic childhood stress. It is also a beautiful book about hope and healing.

Adverse Childhood Experiences (ACEs) are rightly considered a colossal global epidemic and our greatest unaddressed public health problem. ACEs are causally linked to an extremely wide array of psychological, medical, social, spiritual, and functional problems in adults. Nearly everyone is affected by ACEs, either directly or indirectly through loved ones. And the wounds from toxic childhood stress, if unhealed, are often passed from generation to generation.

Beyond the enormous human suffering they cause, ACEs cost the American economy alone trillions of dollars annually from healthcare, welfare, criminal justice, special education, premature mortality, and lost economic productivity.

The first research linking ACEs to a wide range of harmful health outcomes was published in 1998. Since that time, numerous studies have consistently confirmed that link, and added to the list of health conditions caused by ACEs. Despite this important research, the ACEs epidemic remains a silent one, often unrecognized. As the pioneering researcher Vincent Felitti, MD observed, we focus on the downstream smoke (health conditions resulting from ACEs that range from depression, suicide, and drug abuse to obesity, cancer, and heart disease), but fail to address the causal flame of ACEs.

Michael Menard is an extraordinary individual, uniquely qualified to be a spokesperson for the movement to eradicate this silent epidemic. Menard himself is a survivor of multiple ACEs, and writes from very personal, lived experience. He grew up in a 900-square-foot home, below the poverty line, and was one of fourteen children facing uncommon challenges. While most of his siblings attained exceptional success in athletics, their occupations, and their families, many also faced struggles and carried hidden wounds from their childhood adversities—including two deaths from drug overdoses, divorces, and health problems.

In meeting his childhood challenges, Menard forged extraordinary resilience. In so many ways, he rose above the force that is "greater than gravity"—the heavy weight that burdens so many ACEs survivors. Menard's parents were a study in contrasts, a devil on one shoulder and an angel on the other. His mother was a loving, kind woman who cherished each of her children, and taught them to love and forgive all people, including their father. Menard's father was violent, critical, hard as nails, known as a brawler and "badass" for miles around. Highlighting the intergenerational cycle of ACEs, Menard's grandfather was a mean alcoholic who regularly beat his son and took him as a teen to bars for bare-knuckled fights against grown men. Menard's father worked three jobs to support his family, and so, was largely absent. Yet Menard figured out how to incorporate the valuable lessons from his parents—his mother's kindness and compassion; his father's work ethic and grit—while discarding negative examples.

Being largely unsupervised gave Menard the opportunity and freedom to be creative. He discovered a way to make gloves from the skins of the mice that infested the house. Based on his experience babysitting his siblings, Menard came up with the idea of disposable diapers with elasticized legs. He shared his idea with Johnson & Johnson, leading to the first of fourteen patents that revolutionized the absorbent products industry. Lacking any technical education, he rose to worldwide vice president of engineering for the company. After departing from Johnson & Johnson, he founded a successful consulting company that helped large organizations better achieve their goals.

Despite health concerns, he figured out how to become a happy adult and could have retired to a life of ease. And then something transformative happened—he began writing his memoir, *The Kite that Couldn't Fly: And Other May Avenue Stories*. The book began as a series of entertaining bedtime stories for his young children. Yet he cried for some of his siblings. *Why*, he thought, *did some thrive in so many ways, while others stumbled?* He decided to devote his skills and energies to help his siblings and others who had similarly suffered.

As he tried to better understand the complexities of difficult childhoods, a mental health professional introduced him to my book, *The Adverse Childhood Experiences Recovery Workbook*. Shortly thereafter, Michael contacted me and we arranged to meet. We have since spent many hours discussing ACEs, the problems they present, and their solutions. I am extremely grateful our paths crossed so unexpectedly and that I am now privileged to call Michael my colleague and friend. I quickly discerned that Michael is an unusually gifted individual with an expansive mind and the ability to connect concepts from diverse disciplines. His corporate experience has helped him hone his talent for turning useful ideas into practical solutions and applying them on a large scale.

He is also a warm, earnest man who sincerely wishes to end ACEs. The concern he has felt for his siblings now extends to all who have been wounded by ACEs. He has tirelessly devoted himself to studying, interviewing, and making sense of the complexities of childhood trauma and, when unresolved, its long-term effects on adults.

His heartfelt desire to help others led him to start a foundation dedicated to healing the wounds from toxic childhood stress and ultimately eradicating ACEs. His dream is to provide free therapy for those affected by ACEs.

As only a passionate person who has "been there" can, in *Greater than Gravity: How Childhood Trauma is Pulling Down Humanity*, Michael eloquently explains how ACEs wound the mind, body, and spirit, and offers fresh and powerful ideas for treating and preventing the damage caused by ACEs. In his writing, his gift as master storyteller brings a touch of humanity to the stark and cold statistics of ACEs.

I am grateful Michael has written this remarkable book. I know that it will inform, inspire, and help many people—those who have survived ACEs, those who care about affected loved ones, and those who desire to prevent the enormous suffering caused by the silent ACEs epidemic.

–Glenn R. Schiraldi, PhD., LTC US Army (ret.)
Stress Management Faculties at the Pentagon, University
of Maryland, and the International Critical Incident
Stress Foundation
Author of *The Adverse Childhood Experiences Recovery
Workbook*; *The Post-Traumatic Stress Disorder Sourcebook*;
The Resilience Workbook; *The Self-Esteem Workbook*

Tangible: Something that is perceptible by touch or capable of being touched; having actual physical substance or material form. The word can also be used more broadly to describe something that is real, concrete, or substantial, as opposed to something abstract or intangible.

Contagion: The spread of a harmful or undesirable phenomenon, such as a disease, emotion, or ideas among individuals and/or groups. In the context of diseases, contagion refers to the transmission of an illness from one person to another through direct or indirect contact. Contagion can lead to rapid escalation in the number of affected individuals if not properly managed.

Global Health Crisis

Unseen Threat Originating in Childhood, Erupting in Adulthood

THIS IS A SPECIAL breaking news report. We have received alarming information regarding a newly discovered contagion, now believed to be the world's greatest unaddressed public health threat. Recent findings indicate that over 4 billion people across the globe have been infected with this contagion, with an estimated 180 million individuals in the United States affected. Tragically, experts project that an astonishing 11.4 million of them will die 20 years too early due to complications associated with this disease. Those infected are 9.5 times more likely to attempt suicide.

This contagion poses a unique threat as it can only be transmitted to children under the age of 18. Those who contract it may not immediately experience adverse effects, but they are at a significant risk of developing serious mental and metabolic illness decades later. In fact, it is already responsible for contributing to 20 million reported cases of depression among adults in the United States alone.

The financial implications of this contagion are staggering. Treatment costs for associated illnesses and disorders could reach an astounding $14.1 trillion per year, which includes losses from decreased productivity. Exposure to this contagion also appears to dramatically increase high risk and criminal behavior. Alarmingly, data shows that 95% of all adults currently incarcerated in the United States were exposed to this contagion as children, highlighting its far-reaching impact on communities and society at large.

Exposure to this contagion in childhood is apparently responsible for a dramatic increase in the likelihood of biomedical disease years and decades later. Exposure can increase the probability of heart disease by 150%, liver disease by 202%, and likelihood of a stroke by 158%. While exposure to the contagion makes some people sick, it makes other people want to die by increasing the probability of attempted suicide.

When a child is exposed to the contagion, it escalates the likelihood of them facing addiction, suicide, and incarceration in adulthood. What was once seen as a public health issue now seems to be self-medication attempts by those affected.

Public health officials urge parents, caregivers, and educators to be vigilant and monitor for signs of developmental changes in children, as early intervention may be critical. Measures to contain and manage this affliction are being urgently discussed at local, state, and federal levels.

We will continue to provide updates as more information becomes available. Remember to stay safe and informed. For now, we return to our regular programming, but please remain vigilant regarding this developing story.

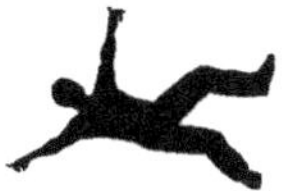

While the announcement you just read may be fictitious, it's all based on truth, one that is deeply rooted in data and science.

The alarming nature of that message is emblematic of the very real crisis that is childhood trauma—a pervasive issue that truly is pulling down humanity. The statistics presented are based on actual findings from global studies, demonstrating that the effects of childhood trauma remain severe, regardless of whether they are widely acknowledged. Childhood trauma is a tangible contagion in the sense that its impacts ripple outwards, affecting not just those who endure it but also their families, communities, and societies. It contributes to a range of mental health challenges, physical health issues, and social dysfunctions that can span generations and is almost impossible to overstate.

My hope with *Greater than Gravity: How Childhood Trauma is Pulling Down Humanity* is to evoke a sense of urgency—an understanding that we cannot afford to look away from or dismiss the reality before us. Childhood trauma is not just an individual concern; it is a systemic issue that has the potential to interfere with societal progress and well-being.

*"Buried beneath the weight of society's progress lies
a silent epidemic: the profound and lasting impact of
childhood trauma, a force that not only shatters individual
lives but threatens the very foundation of our collective
humanity—a force greater than gravity."*

Introduction

In a world that prides itself on being the most health-conscious society in history, we find ourselves facing a troubling paradox: Despite our obsession with wellness, our collective health is on the decline. The wellness industry thrives and profits from our relentless determination to eat better, age gracefully, and feel vibrant. We are bombarded by a constant stream of health headlines, advertising, and trending online content, each promoting the latest self-improvement craze. In our efforts to achieve optimal health, we embrace supplements, enroll in fitness classes, experiment with various diets, invest in genetic assessments, and seek both conventional and alternative treatments for an array of ailments that plague our bodies and minds.

Yet, despite these endeavors, we are witnessing a rise in chronic diseases, mental health disorders, and substance abuse. This begs the question: What is happening? How is it that in an age marked by unparalleled medical advancements and knowledge, we are confronted with escalating health issues that affect both our physical and mental well-being? More perplexingly, how can we remain so unfazed by—or even unaware of—this decline?

As I completed this book, I made a discovery so shocking it stopped me in my tracks. Hidden in plain sight within government data lies proof that childhood trauma is killing 1,401 Americans every day. Its lethality makes childhood trauma the leading cause of death in the United States, exceeding even tobacco.[1] We've been counting the bodies wrong. When someone with severe childhood trauma dies of a heart attack at 55 instead of 75, we record it as heart disease. When they overdose, it's addiction. When they take their own life, it's suicide. But these aren't separate epidemics—they're symptoms of the same hidden crisis that's been destroying lives for generations.

The numbers are staggering and irrefutable. Among the 11.4 million Americans who experienced six or more ACEs, every single one will die 20 years too soon.[2] A crushing 89.4% of teen suicide attempts trace back to adverse childhood experiences,[3] while 85-100% of addiction patients have trauma histories.[4] This isn't just a health crisis—it's an economic catastrophe costing America $14 trillion annually, roughly 60% of our entire GDP.[5] That's more than we spend on defense, education, and infrastructure combined. We're hemorrhaging lives—and resources—to an enemy we refuse to name.

Most shocking of all, this epidemic claims our children, too. Every single day, nine children under 18 die from trauma-related causes—five from homicide, mostly at the hands of their own parents, and four from suicide.[6]

These aren't just statistics. These are Patrick and Adam, my brothers who died from drug overdoses. These are millions of Americans, paralyzed by forces greater than gravity. This book proves childhood trauma isn't just a personal tragedy—it's the greatest threat to humanity itself.

As we embark on this journey to explore the impact of childhood trauma—a foundational element in understanding our current health crisis—I invite you to join me in seeking answers. Together, we will investigate the roots of the problem and uncover the intricate relationship between unresolved trauma and the deteriorating health of our society.

Childhood trauma casts a long shadow over the human experience, and much of the pervasive sadness, loneliness, depression, anxiety, addiction, crime, and illness that afflict our society can be traced to its often-hidden wounds. Though we term it "childhood trauma" because it begins with adverse experiences during those formative years, the fallout extends far beyond childhood itself. The devastation initiated in youth ripples into adulthood, leaving some to grapple with its consequences for a lifetime. This insidious cycle, coupled with its staggering prevalence, reveals childhood trauma to be a profound threat to the very fabric of humanity.

In my advanced years, I have discovered life is a continuous journey of transformation, where every ending becomes a beginning, every challenge becomes a lesson, and every moment of change reveals the endless potential within us all. My journey has given me a radically different perspective on the story of childhood adversity—the complete story, not just the story you think you know. As you read on, you will better understand how childhood adversity may be playing out in your life or in the life of someone you love. What's more important, you will understand the promise of healing, and while that begins with one person or one community, this healing has the power to transform the health of all of humanity.

I feel an ever-present force that is greater than gravity in our world, fractured by childhood trauma, and by all the quiet corners of our past, where memories and hidden wounds reside. Despite this force, I also have an unwavering confidence that ahead lies the powerful promise for transformation. That's exactly what I seek to unravel through this book.

The seed for writing *Greater Than Gravity* was planted in the middle of writing my memoir, *The Kite That Couldn't Fly: And Other May Avenue Stories* released in June of 2024. I am the second eldest of 14 children, all from the same parents, no twins. My siblings and I grew up in a 900-square-foot home located at 118 South May Avenue in Kankakee, Illinois. We lived below the poverty line with a wonderful mother and a father with a PhD in Badassery, shaped by his own childhood trauma. In this memoir, I shared my true childhood stories that in many ways are grander than fiction.

When writing the stories—many sad and clearly depicting suffering—I tried convincing myself they didn't happen. I had a hard time believing and reliving the sadness. Halfway through writing *The Kite That Couldn't Fly*, I sought advice from mental health professionals. Not for therapy for myself, rather to better understand if there were learnings from my childhood I could share with my readers. I cast a wide net, speaking with psychologists, psychiatrists, and therapists and reading more than thirty books about childhood trauma.

Yes, I had gone down a rabbit hole. I began experiencing feelings foreign to me: confusion and a constant thread of sadness, much like depression. From over 350 research reports, I learned that somewhere between 64% and 85% of all adults have experienced childhood trauma. I learned about the disintegration and destruction that begins within a child when exposed to toxic trauma. I also learned the first step in healing from childhood trauma is to revisit and face what happened, even when it's hard. These types of memories become fragmented and buried, making it difficult to make sense of what happened.

I continued to grieve and cry. Not for myself, but for my siblings and for all those who have and are experiencing complex childhood trauma. I eventually stopped grieving and began writing. I climbed out of the hole, brushed myself off, and finished my book.

After publishing *The Kite That Couldn't Fly*, I remained consumed by my newfound knowledge about the devastation and prevalence of childhood trauma. I continued to read and research, which often led me to the works of Dr. Glenn Schiraldi, who I now see as the authority on Post Traumatic Stress Disorder (PTSD), childhood trauma recovery, and resilience. Dr. Schiraldi has become a friend and colleague and has heavily influenced the writing of this very book.

Here is a summary of what I have learned:

When a child is exposed to toxic trauma, the impact is cataclysmic—almost beyond belief. The destruction and disorders toxic trauma create, when left untreated, forge pathways for mental and physical illness that extend well into adulthood. Indeed, the prevalence of childhood trauma may well be called the number one unaddressed public health concern in the world today, leaving devastating consequences in its wake. I've witnessed this firsthand in a family of 14 children, whose spectrum of trauma-induced disorders proved to be a microcosm of the destruction documented across all of humanity—making this crisis both deeply personal and real.

While pockets of excellent work that address this issue do exist, no one has yet connected all the dots or sounded the alarm for this global crisis. Despite being extensively scanned, diagnosed, and medicated, true healing from childhood trauma remains elusive. The United States has a proud history of successfully addressing major public health challenges, from ensuring clean water to combating polio, measles, cancer, HIV, and tobacco-related deaths. Yet remarkably, there has never been a unified, concerted effort to understand, reduce, or eliminate the devastation caused by childhood trauma.

It is time to hit the panic button, and I raise my hand high to do so.

Greater Than Gravity is more than just a title; it is intended to capture the profound impact and monumental challenge that eradicating childhood trauma presents. This issue is an extraordinary force, one that surpasses the fundamental laws we are familiar with, much like the pervasive influence of trauma that grips not only individuals, but all of humanity.

With *Greater Than Gravity*, I now say loudly and proudly: This *is* a call to action. While I offer the disclaimer that I am not a therapist, nor a mental or physical illness expert, I do believe I have the ability and opportunity to offer help and hope given my life's and my siblings' experiences. In this book, I will share what I now know to be the best current practices and healing interventions. In this regard, I see myself as a conduit.

This is a guide for varied audiences and readers who seek to shift the archetype of how we engage with, support, and ultimately heal from the scars left by adverse childhood experiences (ACEs). *Greater Than Gravity* is aimed at three distinct groups:

The first are those who suffer directly from the destruction created by childhood trauma. For these people, *Greater Than Gravity* offers hope and a pathway to healing. Most importantly, I want survivors to know they are not alone in their pain.

The second group includes those living with or close to the sufferers of childhood trauma—partners, friends, family members, or caregivers. Understanding the complexities of trauma is crucial for this group, as their role can significantly influence the recovery process. All the experts agree: Love is the secret sauce. It's not the only ingredient needed, but it's the most important.

Lastly, this book addresses a broader audience—those who, upon understanding the crisis of childhood trauma, feel called and compelled to contribute to a collective solution. This group includes educators, healers, policymakers, community leaders, and anyone with a desire to activate real change.

These three groups encompass virtually every adult on the planet.

I've written this book with great expectations, driven by a profound vision for change. My hope is that *Greater Than Gravity* will serve as a powerful catalyst, compelling the world to look directly at childhood trauma and confront its devastating reality. Consider this both a comprehensive guide for healing and a rallying cry for action—in which I offer practical strategies, expert insights, and personal narratives that illustrate real, human experiences and foster hope and resilience.

Greater Than Gravity is an invitation to join a movement—a call for unity in addressing one of humanity's greatest unspoken crises. By understanding childhood trauma's true impact, implementing effective interventions, and committing to prevention, we can forge a path toward healing that extends from individuals to entire communities. Ultimately, *Greater Than Gravity* is a testament to the capacity of the human spirit to overcome even the most profound adversities and champions a collective movement toward a healthier, more compassionate world.

You may find this book's contents troubling and shocking. It may even be disturbing—and it should be. The problem we face begs for a solution. I hope this book creates a ripple effect that ends the suffering of literally billions of people around the globe. If you or someone you love is affected by childhood trauma, this book will change your life, too.

Let us create the counterforce that is greater than gravity.

Book I

The Crisis

Childhood trauma is the hidden epidemic that weighs heavily on the hearts and minds of billions of individuals, leaving scars that often linger long into adulthood. In The Crisis, we will dissect the multifaceted nature of childhood trauma, starting with a clear definition of what it is—and what it is not.

First, we will reveal the nuances of this complex issue, dispelling common misconceptions that can diminish its importance and impact. From there, we will explore how exposure to trauma alters a child's developing mind and body, which reshapes their perceptions, behaviors, and even their biology. This lays the groundwork for our examination of the long-lasting consequences, where we will confront the destruction and disintegration wrought by childhood trauma, how it may make people mentally and physically sick, and how it even makes some want to die.

Finally, we will confront the sobering reality of the prevalence of childhood trauma across all of humanity. Let me be very clear: this crisis is not confined to specific demographics. Rather, it is a universal challenge that manifests in varying locations from places as remote as Amazonia to main street America, resulting in mental, physical, social, and spiritual disintegration that is pulling down individuals, their communities, and entire societies.

It is only by confronting this crisis head-on, understanding its roots, and acknowledging its far-reaching consequences that we can begin to heal—not just individuals, but our humanity as a whole.

Join me as we navigate this urgent examination of childhood trauma, for is not just a personal struggle, but a collective burden that we must address as a collective to forge a brighter future for all.

CHAPTER ONE

Maybe We Need a New Mirror

"Because we think in a fragmentary way, we see fragments. And this way of seeing leads us to make actual fragments of the world."

–Susan Griffin, A Chorus of Stones

I fiND MYSELF GRAPPLING with an internal conflict. On one hand, I want to present the facts of this issue with clarity and integrity, adhering to the conventions of academic discourse that guide so much of the literature on childhood trauma. On the other hand, an urgent voice inside me cries out, demanding to be heard: "This is the largest threat to the well-being of humanity known today!"

The shocking destruction from and prevalence of childhood trauma has ignited a passionate fretfulness in me—not just for my own siblings, who carry the invisible wounds of their past, but for the billions of individuals around the globe who are silently suffering. It is a burden that weighs heavily on my heart. Each statistic represents not just a number but a story; each case of trauma echoes through generations, leaving its mark on families and communities, on all of us.

How can I write about something so profound and pervasive without allowing my emotions to seep into these pages? How can I convey the reality of this widespread issue without sounding alarmist or overly dramatic? How do I not sound like "the sky is falling!" or "wolf, wolf!"? Yet, the truth is undeniable: the impacts of childhood trauma ripple outward, affecting mental health, relationships, and societal structures in ways that demand our attention and action.

My aim is not just to inform, but to rather awaken a collective awareness. This topic is not merely an academic concern; it is a human one that warrants our deepest respect and our most earnest engagement. As we journey through the layers of complexity and often painful topic of childhood trauma, I invite you to please keep at the top of your mind that the statistics I share reflect real lives. Childhood trauma is not just a personal struggle; it is a public health crisis that beckons us to act with compassion, understanding, and most important of all, urgency.

Before we go any further, I must address what I believe is the reason childhood trauma has gone largely unaddressed in our society: fragmentation.

We are taught from a young age to focus on the pieces, to break things down to their most basic elements, into fragments. We are comfortable with pieces. When we attempt to view and understand the whole, we become overwhelmed and retreat to the comfortable few pieces we understand. This gives us a sense of control, and we surrender our attempts to look at the whole of the issue.

This fragmentation mirrors a profound truth about trauma itself. When children experience trauma, their memories can shatter like a broken mirror, scattering into pieces that become difficult to reassemble. The brain, protecting itself from overwhelming pain, stores these fragments in different corners of consciousness, making it challenging to see the complete picture of the experience. Just as we struggle to view society's challenges holistically, trauma survivors often struggle to piece together their own histories.

David Bohm, one of the most significant physicists of the 20th century, dedicated his life to making major contributions to quantum theory, philosophy of the mind, and the concept of wholeness. Bohm said given our human cognitive limitations, trying to view the whole is futile, almost impossible.[7] This can be compared to attempts to view the whole as trying to put back the pieces of a broken mirror to get a true reflection; think Humpty Dumpty.

Maybe we need a new mirror—both as a society and as individuals healing from trauma.

For society, understanding the whole of childhood trauma isn't just important, it is required to begin the journey to end this crisis. We need a better vantage point. Lucky for us, there are systems available to us that greatly extend our view. Data collection, synthesis, visualization, and communication open the mind to new insights and discovery; clear and precise information leads to clear and precise thinking. Imagine the powerful benefits we might generate if we could connect the dots between all the pockets of knowledge and research surrounding childhood trauma. The problem is that currently, in most cases, these pockets are researched and targeted individually.

For individuals, healing often begins with the painstaking work of gathering these fragments of memory, understanding they need not remain forever broken. Just as we require new tools and perspectives to see the full scope of childhood trauma in society, survivors need support and understanding to reassemble their fragmented memories into a coherent narrative that can finally be faced, processed, and ultimately, transcended.

Let me be clear: Healing from childhood trauma requires us to face a complex truth. If you experienced abuse, neglect, or other adverse childhood experiences (ACEs), you were indeed a victim of circumstances beyond your control. Traumatic experiences are not your fault. The responsibility lies with those who inflicted the trauma, whether they intended harm or were themselves acting from their own wounded places.

However, recognizing past victimization doesn't mean you must remain a victim. The journey from "I was a victim" to "I am a survivor" begins with acknowledging what happened and ends with choosing not to let bitterness and blame define your future. This isn't about digging up dirt on parents or offenders, nor is it about harboring anger that could poison your own healing. Instead, it's about understanding that while you couldn't control what happened to you as a child, you now have the power to shape your path forward.

Let this serve as our new mirror, so we may recognize the full scope of childhood trauma, and also as a gentle guide for survivors piecing together their own fragmented reflections. As we connect the dots that reveal the true scale of this crisis, may survivors find the support and understanding needed to reconstruct their own narrative. The journey to healing requires honesty—both about what happened and about how one chooses to move forward. Using trauma as an excuse for harmful behavior only extends its power over your life. Sometimes, that first step is as simple as opening up to someone you trust and love, saying, "This happened to me," and "I'm ready to move beyond it."

CHAPTER TWO

Drawing the Line
What is Childhood Trauma?

"Trauma is perhaps the most avoided, ignored, belittled, denied, misunderstood, and untreated cause of human suffering."

–Peter A. Levine and Maggie Kline, Trauma Through a Child's Eyes

UNCLE JOHN IS SOMEONE you need to know. A retired Colonel from the US Army, he embodies discipline and integrity. His years of service are etched in his stoic demeanor and commanding presence, making him both intriguing and, at times, a bit intimidating without even trying. Despite his formidable exterior, those who know him well appreciate his unwavering dedication to his principles and genuine kindness. His conversations, rich with stories and insights from life and his military career, offer a glimpse into a life marked by commitment and honor, leaving a lasting impression on all who have the privilege of knowing him. A true gentleman, Uncle John's influence extends beyond his achievements, as he consistently inspires those around him to pursue excellence and uphold the values he holds dear.

It was my first visit to Uncle John and Aunt Cheryl's since the release of my book, *The Kite That Couldn't Fly*. I predicted that Uncle John had not read my book. Hours into our visit, Uncle John looked sideways at me.

"How's the book doing?" Over the years, I had learned that Uncle John prefers short answers—just the facts, please. True to form, John followed up with a very specific question. "In one sentence, define childhood trauma."

One sentence? I had just used 83,000 words describing the subject. I thought about negotiating for three sentences, then quickly realized the futility of that idea.

"Any action against a child up to age 18 that has negative long-lasting psychological, emotional, and physiological effects," I replied. I took the risk of adding, "Not talking about a disappointment like not getting that new bike. I'm talking about neglect, abuse and or growing up in a household with the dysfunction of addiction, separation, or mental illness."

Uncle John showed me grace by not asking if I could count. A subtle nod signaled that Uncle John understood and agreed with my definition.

Allow me to go a bit deeper than one sentence definitions. Throughout this book, I will use the terms childhood trauma and Adverse Childhood Experiences (ACEs) to mean the same thing. Other names for childhood trauma included toxic stress, childhood abuse, and molestation.

Let's start by thinking of childhood trauma and adverse childhood experience as an event. In his book *Trauma Through a Child's Eyes*, Dr. Peter Levine defines childhood trauma as "any experience that stuns us like a bolt out of the blue; it overwhelms us, leaving us altered and disconnected from our bodies. Any coping mechanisms we may have had are undermined and we feel utterly helpless and hopeless. It's as if our legs are knocked out from under us."

The term Adverse Childhood Experiences (which I'll often refer to as ACEs) is now widely accepted and used by the mental and physical health communities. ACEs are possible traumatic events that occur from birth through age 17. ACEs came to fruition through a study conducted by Dr. Vincent Felitti and Dr. Robert Anda to identify negative critical conditions a child may experience and their lasting impacts. Dr. Felitti, the head of Kaiser Permanente's Department of Preventive Medicine in San Diego, along with Dr. Anda, a researcher for the Centers for Disease Control and Prevention, performed a study between 1995–1997 with the hypothesis that childhood trauma is relational to poor physical and mental health in adults. The two doctors collected survey data from 17,421 patients, which was gathered during the patients' physical exams. The adverse childhood experience survey consisted of 10 questions to identify traumas and neglect experienced before the age of 18, and each question was an ACE. The ACEs were identified as neglect (emotional or physical), abuse (sexual, emotional, or physical), and household dysfunctions including parental divorce or separation, domestic violence, incarceration, substance abuse and addiction, and mental health problems.

The results of the study were shocking. There was a direct connection and correlation between a child experiencing ACEs and poor mental and physical well-being as an adult.[8]

The adverse childhood experience survey is now the most widely used tool to score an individual's ACEs. Respondents answer "yes" or "no" to each question, and the total score reflects the number of adverse experiences a person experienced in childhood. The maximum score for the survey is a 10. The 10 questions included in the ACEs survey are as follows.

1. **Emotional Abuse:** Did a parent or other adult in the household often or very often swear at you, put you down, or humiliate you? Or act in a way that made you afraid that you might be physically hurt?

2. **Physical Abuse:** Did a parent or other adult in the household often or very often push, grab, slap, or throw something at you? Or sometimes hurt you physically?

3. **Sexual Abuse:** Did an adult or person at least five years older than you often or very often touch or fondle you or have you touch their body in a sexual way? Or attempt or have oral, anal, or vaginal intercourse with you?

4. **Emotional Neglect:** Did you often or very often feel that no one in your family loved you or thought you were important or special? Or that your family didn't look out for each other, feel close to each other, or support each other?

5. **Physical Neglect:** Did you often or very often feel that your parents or caregivers didn't provide enough food, clothing, or shelter? Or that they were too drunk or high to take care of you or take you to the doctor if you needed it?

6. **Household Dysfunction:** Did a household member go to prison?

7. **Substance Abuse:** Did a household member often or very often feel that your parents or caregivers were too drunk or high to take care of you or take you to the doctor if you needed it?

8. **Mental Illness:** Did a household member often or very often suffer from a mental illness, or attempt suicide, or have a mental illness that made life difficult for you?

9. **Parental Separation or Divorce:** Were your parents ever separated or divorced?

10. **Domestic Violence:** Did a parent or other adult in the household often or very often push, grab, slap, or throw something at your other

parent? Or sometimes or often hit the other so hard that they had injuries?

The original ACEs study by Drs. Felitti and Anda was indeed a landmark discovery, shining a crucial light on the profound effects of childhood trauma on long-term health and well-being. However, it is important to note that it focused primarily on adverse experiences that occurred within the household and was conducted largely with middle-class populations. These limitations left out a broader range of potential childhood traumas that can significantly impact a child's development and mental health.

In addition to the types of traumas assessed in the original ACEs survey—such as emotional and physical abuse, neglect, and household dysfunction—there are several other external threats that can contribute to childhood adversity, including:

11. **Community Violence:** Exposure to violence in the neighborhood, such as gun violence, gang activity, or physical assault.
12. **Bullying:** Experiences of bullying, whether in-person or online, that can lead to emotional distress and social isolation.
13. **Discrimination:** Experiences of racism, homophobia, transphobia, or other forms of discrimination that can affect a child's sense of safety and self-worth.
14. **Natural Disasters:** Traumatic experiences related to natural disasters such as hurricanes, earthquakes, and fires that impact a child's sense of security.
15. **Socioeconomic Instability:** Experiencing poverty, homelessness, or instability in living conditions, creating chronic stress and insecurity.

16. **Parental Substance Abuse:** While the original ACEs survey addresses household dysfunction, the implications of parental substance abuse on broader family dynamics and external environments are significant.

17. **Childhood Illness or Disability:** Experiencing a serious illness or disability, either personally or within the family, can impose stress and trauma that affects a child's well-being.

18. **Loss of a Parent or Caregiver:** Bereavement due to death or estrangement can profoundly affect a child's emotional stability.

By acknowledging these additional forms of trauma, we can gain a more comprehensive understanding of childhood adversity and its consequences, ultimately allowing for more effective interventions and support systems for children affected by a wider range of traumatic experiences.

If a child has experienced any one or more of these 18 types of traumas, we can say that child has experienced childhood trauma. However, there are additional trauma definitions that deserve attention: complex trauma, complex post-traumatic stress disorder (C-PTSD), and secondary trauma.

Complex Childhood Trauma refers to prolonged or repeated exposure to traumatic events during childhood—particularly those that occur within the context of caregiving relationships or home environments. Unlike single-event traumas, complex traumas typically involve a series of traumatic experiences that can have a cumulative and compounding effect on the child. The Georgetown University Center for Child and Human Development explains that complex trauma is chronic, begins in childhood, and occurs within the primary caregiving environment. The original ACEs study reports that if a child experiences one ACE, that child has an 87% chance to experience more ACEs.

Complex Post-Traumatic Stress Disorder (C-PTSD) is a psychological condition that can develop in individuals who have experienced complex trauma during their formative years. While it shares characteristics with standard trauma, C-PTSD includes additional symptoms and challenges that are distinctively related to the nature of prolonged exposure to trauma.

Secondary trauma, also known as vicarious trauma or compassion fatigue, refers to the emotional and psychological impact experienced by individuals who are indirectly exposed to the traumatic experiences of others, particularly in the context of childhood trauma and ACEs. This phenomenon often affects siblings of the child being traumatized as well as caregivers, educators, healthcare professionals, social workers, and first responders who work closely with children who have faced trauma.

Adult trauma and childhood trauma differ in several keyways, including their origins, the developmental context in which they occur, the psychological implications, and the coping mechanisms often employed by individuals affected by each. While adult trauma can be just as serious and devastating, I have a single-minded focus for this book: childhood trauma.

Childhood is rife with challenge and disappointment, which should generally lead to important lessons and opportunities for growth. This is a great thing, but it's essential to differentiate between genuine childhood trauma—adverse childhood experiences (ACEs) that can have profound and lasting psychological effects—and experiences that may be difficult or disappointing but do not constitute trauma in a clinical sense. I've compiled a list of items or experiences that someone might incorrectly label as childhood trauma.

1. **Not getting desired material possessions:** As mentioned in my Uncle John story, not being able to get expensive sneakers, toys, or gadgets that peers have can be disappointing for a child, but it usually doesn't qualify as trauma.

2. **Minor disagreements with peers:** Experiencing a common childhood argument with friends or peers, such as quarrels over games or toys, is typical and usually does not rise to the level of trauma.

3. **Missing out on extracurricular activities:** Not being allowed to participate in a particular sport or club due to scheduling conflicts or parental restrictions can be frustrating but does not constitute trauma.

4. **Temporary geographic relocation:** Moving to a new city or neighborhood can be challenging and may cause anxiety, but a single relocation that doesn't involve threats to safety or stability is typically not traumatic.

5. **Household rules or discipline:** Experiencing strict rules or disciplinary actions from parents or guardians might feel unfair, but it's part of normal parenting unless it escalates into abusive behavior.

6. **Academic pressure:** Feeling stressed about grades or performance in school is common and does not equate to trauma unless associated with severe, ongoing anxiety or distress resulting from abuse or extreme expectations.

7. **Being ignored or overlooked in social settings:** Feeling excluded from a group at school or not receiving enough attention at a party can be hurtful, but typically it does not rise to the level of trauma.

8. **Experiencing "FOMO" (Fear of Missing Out):** The feeling of missing out on parties, trends, or experiences, while distressing, is a normal part of growing up and does not constitute trauma.

9. **Sibling rivalry:** Normal competition or conflict between siblings might lead to feelings of jealousy or frustration, but these are typical experiences that usually do not represent trauma.

10. **Having different interests from peers:** Feeling like an outcast for having unique hobbies or tastes is disappointing but is often a part of healthy social development rather than trauma.

11. **Parental separation during activities:** Experiencing a temporary separation from a parent during an outing or event may cause momentary distress but is usually not traumatic unless the context is abusive or neglectful.

12. **Not receiving a reward or recognition:** Failing to win an award or receive recognition in school or sports, while disappointing, does not represent trauma.

13. **Participating in minor accidents or injuries:** Experiencing common childhood scrapes or bumps, such as falling off a bicycle, is a part of growing up and typically isn't classified as trauma unless there is major injury accompanied by fear or lasting psychological impact.

These everyday disappointments and challenges absolutely create stress for children, and that stress matters. A failed test, losing a game, or conflict with friends can feel enormous in a child's world. The key difference is that these experiences, while difficult, don't fundamentally threaten a child's sense of safety or disrupt their core development when handled with care and support.

However, context changes everything. If a child is already experiencing true ACEs—living with abuse, neglect, or household dysfunction—these smaller stresses can build up, like rocks in an already-heavy backpack. A fight with a sibling becomes harder to bounce back from when home doesn't feel safe. A disappointment at school affects an elementary schooler differently when there's chaos at home. This is exactly why love, understanding, and guidance from parents and caregivers matter so much. Every interaction is a chance to add to a child's stress or help them build the resilience they'll need to heal and thrive.

It's essential to approach the topic of trauma with care, understanding that while experiences like the aforementioned can be challenging, they do not typically result in the profound psychological consequences associated with true trauma. Acknowledging the difference helps keep our focus on the serious mental health concerns discussed in this book that require attention and care.

Having defined childhood trauma as a detrimental experience that disrupts a child's developmental trajectory, it is crucial to explore the profound and multifaceted impacts these experiences can have on a child's mental, physical, social, and spiritual well-being. Trauma does not merely exist as an isolated event in a child's life; rather, it establishes a ripple effect that extends far into adulthood, shaping not only individual behavior and emotional responses but also influencing relationships, coping mechanisms, and overall quality of life.

Let's explore how these traumatic experiences manifest in various aspects of a child's existence into adulthood.

CHAPTER THREE

When Laughter Fades

The Result of Childhood Exposure to Toxic Trauma

"In my beginning is my end."

–T.S. Eliot, Four Quartets

TRADITIONALLY, IN CONSTRUCTION, THE cornerstone is the first stone laid, placed at the corner of a building to establish its alignment and integrity. Today, a cornerstone is more than just a physical stone; it represents a fundamental element that serves as the foundation for something greater. As we enter this chapter, I invite you to take a moment to reflect deeply. What follows is not merely a narrative, but a cornerstone of understanding—an essential piece that will help you comprehend the larger picture of childhood trauma and its significance.

In the delicate landscape of a child's developing mind, exposure to trauma can create seismic shifts that create a ripple effect, disturbing both neurological and physical well-being. When a child is exposed to what I have defined as childhood trauma, their brain wiring alters in profound ways, impacting emotions, memory, and behavior.

The delicate balance of neurotransmitters can be disrupted, leading to heightened states of fear or anxiety, while the body may respond with chronic stress signals, manifesting in conditions that persist throughout the entire span of adulthood.

It's time to delve into the interplay of mind and body following exposure to trauma. Then, we'll explore the profound resilience needed to navigate the heavy burdens ACEs impose.

It is with a heavy heart that I approach the next pages of this chapter. The profound effects of childhood trauma on a child's mind, body, soul, and entire future are not just painful to witness, they are unbearable to articulate. Each word carries the weight of countless stories, representing the darkness that can infiltrate a young life and cast long shadows over their journey.

For some readers, this exploration may evoke deep pain, bringing forth emotions and memories best left unexamined. If you find yourself struggling with what you read in the pages to follow, I urge you to set this book aside. Prioritize your well-being—take a break, revisit it later, or choose not to return at all. Your health and healing come first, and it is essential to navigate these difficult waters at your own pace.

When a child is exposed to toxic trauma—whether through neglect, abuse, or family dysfunction—the very fabric of their existence unravels, and nothing will ever be the same. While each child's response to trauma varies based on the type, intensity, and duration of their experiences, certain fundamental changes often occur that can alter the entire trajectory of their lives.

The transformation begins immediately, affecting the child across multiple dimensions.

Physically, their developing brain and body enter a state of hyperarousal—stress hormones flood their system, potentially disrupting normal development and creating lasting changes in how their body responds to stress. The flood of cortisol and other stress hormones damages mitochondria in the brain, a repercussion that can set the stage for mental health disorders. Their immune system may become compromised, and their very DNA can be altered through changes in gene expression.

Mentally, the child's cognitive and emotional development faces severe disruption. Their ability to process information, regulate emotions, and form secure attachments may become impaired. The brain, in its attempt to protect itself, often fragments memories of the trauma, making it difficult for the child to form coherent narratives of their experiences. This fragmentation can persist into adulthood, affecting how they understand and process their past.

Socially, trauma can profoundly impact a child's ability to form and maintain relationships. Trust becomes difficult, and the natural progression of social development may be interrupted. Many children withdraw from peers, struggle with boundaries, or develop maladaptive behaviors in their attempt to navigate a world that suddenly feels unsafe.

Spiritually, trauma can shake a child's fundamental sense of meaning and purpose. Their innate trust in the goodness of the world may be shattered, and their ability to find joy and wonder in life's simple pleasures often diminishes. Some children lose their natural sense of hope and optimism, replacing it with a deep-seated sense of worthlessness or shame.

As the child's brain and body respond to this upheaval, the repercussions can reverberate through their entire lives, potentially manifesting as unhappiness, destructive behaviors, fractured relationships, and a pervasive sense of disintegration. While this book primarily focuses on how these childhood experiences manifest in adulthood, understanding the immediate impact of trauma on children is crucial for recognizing not only the individual suffering but also its far-reaching implications for families, communities, and humanity as a whole.

In Dr. Glenn Schiraldi's book, *The Adverse Childhood Experiences Recovery Workbook*, he writes:

> *"Dis-orders—departures from our usual order—often have multiple causes, such as infection, a toxic physical environment, lack of social support, unhealthy lifestyle, genes, and temperament. However, Felitti and Anda's original study and scores of later studies have shown that ACEs independently predict many disorders and do so in a stepwise fashion. That is, the higher one's ACEs score, the greater the likelihood of developing a disorder."* [9]

The following is a list of the predicted symptoms or outcomes of ACEs, as described by Dr. Schiraldi in his book The Adverse Childhood Experience Recovery Workbook.

Mental Health Conditions: Low self-esteem, depression (including bipolar disorder), anxiety (including panic disorder), post-traumatic stress disorder (PTSD) and complex PTSD, borderline personality disorder, memory disruption, and attention deficit hyperactivity disorder (ADHD)

Medical Conditions: Obesity (eating might self-medicate pain), Type 2 diabetes, cardiovascular disease (heart disease, stroke), cancer, pain, autoimmune diseases (rheumatoid arthritis, Type 1 diabetes, multiple sclerosis, lupus, psoriasis, celiac disease, inflammatory bowel disease, graves' disease, vitiligo, idiopathic pulmonary fibrosis, primary biliary cirrhosis), fibromyalgia, chronic fatigue, hepatitis, nearly all sleep disorders (sleep apnea, nightmares, insomnia, narcolepsy, sleepwalking, sleep eating), reproductive problems (sexually transmitted diseases, preterm birth), ulcers, fractures, shorter life span (by nearly twenty years when ACE score is six or higher) and poorer self-rated health

Social/Risky Behaviors: Drug abuse or misuse (smoking, substance use disorder, injecting drugs intravenously, misusing prescription drugs [taking too much or too often or using them without a prescription, using a higher number of prescriptions]), suicide attempts, precocious sexual activity (greater likelihood of intercourse by age fifteen, having multiple sex partners, teen paternity and maternity, unintended pregnancy), intimate partner violence (greater likelihood of victimization or perpetration, including later being raped), physical inactivity, criminality, occupational or financial challenges (serious problems performing one's job or concentrating, absenteeism, serious financial problems, lower lifetime income), higher number of marriages, and lower educational attainment

How strongly do ACEs predict these conditions? At an ACE score of four or more, compared with zero, the risks typically increase two to five times. The risks are even higher for alcoholism (seven-fold increase), suicide attempts (12-fold increase), and learning and behavioral problems (up to a 33-fold increase for problems including ADHD, which is often misdiagnosed as bipolar disorder).

In addition to disorders and illnesses, those exposed to childhood trauma may experience unnatural and unhealthy emotions and thoughts or other symptoms, including:

Emotional & Physical Arousal

Like a ship tossed in a storm, ACEs create waves that crash through our emotional and physical well-being, destabilizing our sense of safety and calm. This can create difficulty regulating emotions, manifesting as anxiety, including panic attacks, separation anxiety, abandonment fear, and social anxiety; depression; anger; feeling overwhelmed, helpless, or fearful; intolerance of being alone; and difficulty experiencing positive emotions. It can also create a high stress arousal, which could cause an individual to feel on edge, be easily startled, have trouble concentrating or sleeping, or feel either increased irritability, or numb, collapsed, and shut down.

How You Experience Yourself

ACEs can negatively affect our basic sense of self—our identity at the core—in ways that might manifest as:

- Low self-esteem (feeling defective, inadequate, not good enough, unlovable, powerless, helpless)

- Shame, self-loathing, self-contempt

- Feeling emptiness, nothingness, little sense of self

- Feeling that one is not normal

- Feeling dead inside

- Feeling isolated, alienated, alone; rejected, disconnected from others; you don't belong, you are not "at home"

- Lacking confidence in relationships; feeling unworthy or not good enough

Your Worldview

Our deepest wounds often shape the lens through which we see the world, crafting beliefs that once protected us but now hold us back from the connection and security we deserve. Frequent thoughts like these might indicate one's worldview has been affected by ACEs:

- "The world isn't safe."

- "I don't really belong anywhere."

- "Authority figures are frightening or uncomfortable."

- "Relationships are scary."

- "People are not to be trusted or counted on."

Your Coping Methods

The ways we learn to shield ourselves from pain caused by ACEs can become a second skin, creating patterns of behavior that may protect us in the moment but ultimately distance us from authentic connection and growth:

- I am hypersensitive to criticism or rejection.

- I wear a mask of calm that is shaken under intense distress.

- I present a façade of success (I look successful and confident on the outside, while feeling like a mess inside).

- I use extreme, inflexible defenses—self-protecting, keeping others away, extreme independence or letting too many people in (weak boundaries); extreme dependence.

- I am typically dissatisfied with myself or others.

- I compensate for feelings of inadequacy by:

  - Implementing narcissistic behaviors—a façade of superiority that masks vulnerability.

  - Hiding to protect myself—becoming invisible like a shrinking violet; withdrawing from people.

  - Being harshly critical of myself or others.

  - Demanding others' attention (attention that I didn't receive early in life).

  - Perfectionism, overachievement (immoderate pursuit of wealth, being highly competitive, obsessing over one's body image through excessive dieting, body sculpting, etc.)

Pleasing Behavior

If we experienced ACEs, we may have developed intricate ways of surviving that rippled into every aspect of our emotional expression—patterns that, while born of necessity, often linger long after their usefulness has passed. One might be employing pleasing behaviors if they:

- Avoid problems or challenges; give up easily (fearing that one might fail and disappoint self or others).

- Have trouble empathizing (empathy wasn't modeled in the early years).

- Can't tolerate negative or even positive emotions; numbing emotions or concealing feelings for fear that others won't accept or acknowledge them.

- Find it difficult to express emotions with words; instead, emotions are expressed through physical symptoms, such as asthma, diarrhea, infections, skin conditions, pain, collapsing, etc.

- Are overly emotional—often overreacting or becoming dramatic when encountering frustration, disappointments, being ignored, being criticized, etc.

- Suppress or ignore painful feelings; are unaware of their feelings; are overly cerebral or intellectual about their emotions—thinking through their emotions rather than feeling them; deny or avoid unpleasant feelings.

- Have difficulty connecting or cooperating with others.

- Self-medicate emotional pain with substances (drugs seem more dependable than people).

- Harm themself, or risk harm to themself, through drugs, self-injury, casual sex, or other risky behaviors or addictions

Your Posture

If other people were looking at me, they'd likely think that my posture is…

- Rigid (self-protecting)

- Slumped (often seen in people who learned that caregivers won't respond)

Spoken or Unspoken Messages

Shame, abuse, and faulty nurturing in the early years can ingrain messages that are often more felt than thought. As a person matures, these feelings might be expressed in words or unspoken thoughts:

"Something is wrong with me."

"My basic, core self is deeply and permanently damaged."

"I don't matter."

"I'm no good, empty."

"I was treated like trash, so I must be trash."

"I don't belong."

"I displeased my caregiver; therefore, I am unlovable."

"I'm bad."

"I'm powerless, helpless."

"I'm inferior as a person to others."

"I'm defective, worthless."

"The world is dangerous. Something bad is about to happen."

"My feelings don't matter; no one cares what I feel."

"It's uncomfortable to be around people."

"I must be perfect to be loved."

"I'm not enough; I should be more."

"If I'm not perfect, then I'm a loser."

Other Trauma Symptoms

Hidden beneath the surface of our adult lives, ACEs leave their signature in ways both subtle and profound. Additional trauma symptoms include:

- Nightmares, flashbacks, or other intrusive memories. Typically, these are nonverbal, visual, and experienced in the body. These signal that a memory is unprocessed or unsettled.

- A significant change to a previously loving, happy nature. Instead, one might be hypervigilant, easily startled, irritable, or hyperactive.

- State-dependent stress. Stress, or reminders of the stressful past, trigger implicit or explicit memories, along with the initial emotions, sensations, survival impulses, and visceral responses (such as sensations in the gut, heart, chest, throat, or lungs). Thus, being ignored by a significant other might trigger the feeling of being neglected by one's caregiver in the early years. Or a visit home might trigger feelings of inadequacy.

- Dissociation—feeling that you or the world around you is unreal or feeling that you are drifting away from your body or the present when things are stressful.

- Feeling numbness or emotionless.

- Often wearing a blank stare. Sometimes, this is also referred to as a thousand-yard stare or "being somewhere else" mentally.

- Bouncing between extremes. For example: "I'm on top of the world" or "I'm down in the dumps." "My loved one is an angel" or [when he/she disappoints] "My loved one is despicable."

This is an extensive list of disorders, illnesses, negative thoughts, and behaviors that are often associated with childhood trauma. My aim in sharing these is to validate the feelings and experiences of those who may resonate with these symptoms. This list is a resource for identifying potential ramifications that may arise from ACEs. Beyond that, I also want to promote awareness and understanding for those who may not relate to these effects of childhood trauma. Perhaps a reader might recognize the condition in someone they are close to.

While these conditions and negative thought patterns may suggest a history of trauma, it is crucial to remember that their presence does not automatically imply that an individual has experienced childhood trauma. Each person's life journey is unique, and many factors contribute to mental health and well-being.

I encourage everyone to reflect on their own life experiences as they consider the items on this list. Experiencing one or more of these symptoms may point to deeper struggles that could be tied to various life circumstances, including but not limited to childhood trauma. I am confident that if my brother Jamie would have read this chapter twenty-five years ago, he would have saved himself years of ailments and failed efforts trying to find out why he was experiencing depression and anxiety.

Remember, while ACEs affect children the moment they take place—mentally, physically, socially, and spiritually—a person can be affected by their childhood trauma in both profound and subtle ways for the entirety of their adult life.

CHAPTER FOUR

Attachment

"If our society were truly to appreciate the significance of children's emotional ties throughout the first years of life, it would no longer tolerate children growing up, or parents having to struggle, in situations that cannot possibly nourish healthy growth."
–Stanley Greenspan, M.D., The Growth of the Mind

SCIENTIFIC RESEARCH HAS ILLUMINATED the eerie reality that childhood trauma can extend beyond immediate experiences, intertwining with genetic predispositions through a phenomenon known as epigenetics. Incredibly, the effects of stress and trauma can be passed down from parent to child, potentially even manifesting in the womb. This means that a parent's own experiences of trauma can influence the developing brain and biology of their unborn child, setting the stage for a myriad of challenges before the child even takes their first breath. However, for the purpose of this book, I will focus on the starting point as trauma that occurs after birth, as it is during these formative years—amidst relationships, environments, and ongoing experiences—that a child's psychological and emotional landscape is critically shaped.

Attachment between a newborn and their primary caregiver, most often the mother, is a fundamental aspect of healthy child development. This bond serves as the foundation for a child's emotional, social, and cognitive growth, creating a secure base from which they can explore the world around them. The quality of this attachment is largely influenced by the caregiver's responsiveness to the infant's needs—whether through a welcoming smile, physical touch, nurturing, a soothing voice, or consistent care. When a parent unfailingly meets their infant's needs, the child begins to develop a sense of safety and trust, learning that the world can be a reliable and supportive place.

Secure attachment promotes the development of healthy self-esteem, empathy, and resilience, as children internalize the sense of being cared for and valued. Evidence has shown that securely attached children are more likely to exhibit positive social interactions and emotional well-being throughout their lives.

Conversely, when the attachment figure is inconsistent, neglectful, or unresponsive, the child may experience anxiety and insecurity, which can hinder their emotional regulation and social skills.

Disruptions in this pivotal relationship can lead to attachment disorders and various psychological issues, impeding a child's ability to form healthy relationships in the future. When caregivers respond sensitively to their infants' needs, they nurture resilience, empathy, and the ability to form secure relationships later in life. Thus, the attachment formed in these early stages is not merely a protective factor; it lays the groundwork for lifelong development. Attachment influences how individuals navigate relationships, cope with challenges, and ultimately contribute to society. This underscores the critical importance of cultivating this bond from the very beginning.

We feel before we can think. This profound truth, highlighted by researcher and therapist Bruce Perry, Ph.D. underscores why the first sixty days of life are so crucial to human development.[10] During this period, an infant's brain isn't forming thoughts—it's forming *feelings* that will create the foundation for all future emotional responses.

Anthropologist Jean Liedloff makes a key observation: humans spent most of our evolutionary history (all but the last six minutes of an hour-long metaphorical clock) living in small hunter-gatherer groups where child-rearing was communal and connection focused.[11] These societies valued "hospitality, sharing, generosity, and reciprocal exchange," not for personal gain but for collective survival.

Liedloff believes modern society has deviated sharply from this evolutionary blueprint in the past 10,000–15,000 years. Today's culture, as Dr. Stanley Greenspan notes, increasingly disregards "mind-building emotional experiences" in childcare, education, and family life.[12] Social patterns, economic pressures, and cultural imperatives often work against the natural developmental needs of children that evolved over millions of years.

A 2022 study tracking mother-infant pairs over three decades provides compelling evidence: babies who received high levels of maternal affection at eight months showed the lowest levels of emotional distress as adults.[13] Attachment isn't just about feeling loved—it's about building the brain's architecture for handling life's challenges.

A landmark study by Dr. Bruce Perry and other brilliant minds, titled *Beyond the ACE Score: Examining relationships between timing of developmental adversity, relational health and developmental outcomes in children*, shows that what happens to babies in their first 60 days of life has a massive impact on their development and future well-being.[14] The researchers looked at over 3,500 children to understand how early experiences affect brain development. Let me explain the study's key findings.

- The first 60 days are most critical. Lack of nurturing care during this time does more damage than trauma later in childhood.

- Poor emotional connection with caregivers in these early days is actually more harmful than direct trauma or abuse.

- The effects compound over time. Children who had poor early care fell increasingly behind their peers as they grew up.

- Positive relationships later in life can help buffer against early trauma.

The science reveals that emotional neglect in those first 60 days can be more damaging than physical harm. When a parent's face shows chronic distress or lack of engagement, or when they don't respond to their baby's needs for soothing and cuddling, the infant's developing brain interprets this as a threat to survival. Dr. Perry's research found that even subtle signs of maternal disconnection—a flat expression, delayed response to crying, or mechanical rather than loving care—program the baby's neural circuits for chronic stress and fear. This happens because infants can only feel, not think, and their nervous system is exquisitely tuned to read their mother's emotional state. Every unmet cry for connection, every moment without loving touch, every encounter with an unresponsive face rewires their brain's threat detection system.

Emotional neglect in those first 60 days essentially strips away a child's psychological armor, leaving them uniquely vulnerable to future trauma. Further, it's a sad reality that those infants experiencing neglect in the first 60 days are highly likely to experience future ACEs.

The study explains why this happens: newborns are completely dependent on caregivers not just for food and warmth, but for learning how to regulate their emotions and stress responses. When an infant lacks nurturing care during this critical period, their brain's stress response system becomes hypersensitive—like a smoke alarm that blares at the slightest hint of smoke. When these same children later face abuse or trauma, whether from biological or foster parents, the impact is dramatically multiplied because they lack the neural resilience that early nurturing would have provided.

It's as if the neglect in those first 60 days removed their emotional immune system, leaving them with no internal defenses against future psychological wounds. This explains why two children can experience the same traumatic event, yet the child who received loving care in their earliest days often shows more resilience, while the child who faced early neglect may suffer devastating long-term effects.

The researchers emphasize that this isn't about blaming parents—rather, it shows why supporting new mothers and families in those crucial early days should be a top priority for preventing long-term developmental problems.

Case Study 1: Marcy's Cascading Tragedy

At age five, Marcy became a mother to her two-year-old brother while her own mother lay in bed, paralyzed by depression after losing *her* mother in a car accident. In their small apartment, Marcy learned to make cereal, change diapers, and to whisper so she wouldn't wake her mother. Her father's 80-hour work weeks meant financial security, but also absence. When exhaustion shattered his control, his rage filled their home with terror.

By middle school, Marcy's arms told her story in thin white scars. Teachers noted her silence, how she flinched at loud noises, but intervention never came. At 15, she found what felt like love with Tom, age 19. His attention filled the void her parents left empty. Her teenage pregnancy surprised no one who understood trauma's patterns.

Like a dark echo of her mother's depression, Marcy stared at her newborn son without feeling. No one recognized her postpartum depression, no one saw how she propped bottles instead of holding her baby. By 25, she had three children and two failed marriages. Alcohol numbed her pain while prescription pills helped her function. Her children's struggles emerged like clockwork.

- Joey, her oldest, channeled his ADHD and rage into fights by age six.

- Sarah developed such severe anxiety she threw up before school.

- Danny witnessed his father throw Marcy through a glass table and stopped speaking for a year.

The next generation's pain multiplied exponentially.

- Joey's drug dealing led to prison, leaving his own two children in foster care.

- Sarah's own teen pregnancy led to three children of her own by age 20, all showing signs of attachment disorder.

- Danny's untreated trauma manifested as schizophrenia, leading to homelessness.

The mathematical reality of one person's trauma:

- 3 children and five grandchildren directly impacted

- 15 foster families managing traumatized children

- 6 teachers per year adapting classrooms for trauma behaviors

- 8 emergency room visits for domestic violence

- $180,000 annual cost for Danny's untreated mental illness

- $45,000 annual cost for Joey's incarceration

- 12 social workers involved across three generations

- 4 suicide attempts requiring intensive care

- 3 restraining orders involving two different families

- Estimated societal cost: $3.8 million over three generations

One mother's unhealed childhood trauma rippled through generations, creating a devastating human domino effect. Her pain touched over 100 lives directly—children, grandchildren, spouses, teachers, social workers, doctors, police officers—and hundreds more indirectly through overwhelmed systems meant to catch society's falling. Each interaction carried its own cost in dollars, resources, and human potential.

Now just imagine the destruction and disintegration potentially created by the estimated 180 million—the number of adults in the United States *alone*—who carry childhood trauma in their bones. This isn't just about individual tragedy anymore. It's about a society unknowingly engineered to perpetuate cycles of pain. As Dr. Gabor Maté reveals in *The Myth of Normal* that what we label as dysfunction—the addictions, the violence, the mental illness—aren't signs of human brokenness. They're natural responses to profoundly unnatural childhood experiences. When a child's earliest needs for safety and nurturing go unmet, their very biology adapts to survive a world of threat rather than love. Then they grow up, have children of their own, and the cycle continues—not because they're bad parents, but because unhealed wounds bleed across generations.

Every untreated childhood trauma creates new trauma carriers. The cost isn't just measured in dollars spent on prisons, hospitals, and foster care—it's measured in human souls.

Marcy's childhood trauma is an extreme but not an uncommon example of an attachment disorder. More subtle examples of neglect at infancy which we now know initiate stress response dysfunction is depriving the infant from the required responses for the basic needs of food, a dry diaper, nurturing, and love.

There are themes in literature and psychology that explore the impact of a parent's emotional state, particularly a mother's, on a child's development and well-being. One well-known reference is found in the writings of authors and psychologists who discuss attachment theory and the emotional bonds between mothers and their children. One notable book is *The Drama of the Gifted Child* by Alice Miller. Miller discusses how children's happiness and self-worth can be intrinsically tied to their parents' emotional health, especially the mother's. She explores how children may unconsciously carry the emotional burdens of their parents, often leading to feelings of guilt and the feeling they don't deserve to be any happier than their mother.

Our evolutionary history as humans shaped us for close, nurturing connections in our earliest moments of life—a reality that stands in stark contrast to many modern parenting practices. Through groundbreaking research and heartbreaking stories like Marcy's, we now understand that the first 60 days of life represent not just a period of physical development, but a critical window where an infant's nervous system learns whether the world is fundamentally safe or threatening. This biological programming runs deeper than conscious thought, as babies feel before they can think, making early nurturing not just emotionally significant but neurologically essential.

The implications ripple outward like waves in a pond, touching not just individual lives but entire generations. When we understand how early emotional neglect can strip a child's psychological armor—leaving them more vulnerable to future trauma than even direct abuse would—we begin to see why supporting new mothers isn't just a social nicety but a biological imperative. This understanding transforms our perspective from viewing early attachment as simply desirable to recognizing it as fundamentally necessary for human development and societal healing.

CHAPTER FIVE

The Stress Response

"The body keeps the score. The past is alive in the form of gnawing interior discomfort. The body remembers, the bones remember, the joints remember, even the little finger remembers. Memory is loyal to you, and keeps the essence of who you are."

–Dr. Bessel van der Kolk

ONE OF THE MOST significant yet often overlooked consequences of traumatic experiences is their impact on the body's hormonal system.

The human body is amazing. The natural stress response of the mind and body, often referred to as the "fight or flight" response, is an incredible biological mechanism designed to protect us from perceived threats and dangers. This response is rooted in our evolutionary history and is essential for survival.

When we encounter a stressful situation—whether it's a physical danger like a Bigfoot in the woods, an emotional challenge like public speaking, or any other form of stress—our brain quickly assesses the situation and triggers a cascade of physiological changes. Here's how it works:

Perception of Danger: The process begins in the brain, particularly in an area called the amygdala, which is responsible for processing emotions and detecting threats. Once a potential threat is recognized, the amygdala sends a signal to the hypothalamus.

Hormonal Response: The hypothalamus communicates with the adrenal glands, which then release stress hormones such as adrenaline (epinephrine) and cortisol into the bloodstream. These hormones prepare the body to either confront the threat (fight) or flee from it (flight).

Physiological Changes: As cortisol and adrenaline flood the system, a series of physiological changes occur:

- Increased heart rate and blood pressure. This helps pump more blood to vital organs and muscles, preparing the body for rapid action.

- Heightened alertness. The brain becomes more alert and focused, allowing for quicker decision-making and response.

- Redistribution of energy. Energy resources are redirected from non-essential functions (like digestion) to muscles and vital systems necessary for immediate survival.

- Dilation of pupils. This allows more light into the eyes to improve vision and assessment of the environment.

Once the perceived threat is removed, the body gradually returns to a state of balance, or homeostasis. Hormone levels normalize, and physiological processes return to their regular functions.

This stress response is truly amazing because it illustrates how intricately our bodies and minds are designed to work together for our protection. In moments of acute stress, this system can save our life by enabling split-second decisions and actions. Like escaping from that Bigfoot.

However, it's also important to recognize that while this response can be beneficial in the short term, or in life-or-death situations, chronic activation due to ongoing stressors can lead to negative health consequences, including anxiety, depression, and other stress-related disorders.

But what happens when it's not Bigfoot in the woods threatening you? What happens when Bigfoot lives with you?

Case Study 2: Michael's Journey

Michael, my cherished brother-in-law and beloved family member, was a fixture in our lives for nearly 50 years. Married to my sister Mary, he was known for his kind nature, soft-spoken demeanor, and infectious smile. Michael was a devoted husband and father who took great joy in spending time with family, often finding peace sitting on the front porch swing, watching a rainstorm roll in. He was truly one of the good ones, deeply valued by everyone who knew him.

As we became close in our early adulthood, Michael shared his childhood memories with me. Michael's dad was an alcoholic, a mean drunk. When his dad came home, almost always stumble down drunk, his mother would hide young Michael in a large hope chest on the second floor and tell him not to come out until she came to get him. Michael would have to listen to the long and brutal beatings. When there was silence, he always feared his mom was beaten to death, until she would rescue him from the darkness; his mom's face often battered.

Throughout Michael's adult life, Mary noticed that he carried the weight of his childhood experiences. She often suggested he seek professional help or therapy to process his past traumas. Michael consistently refused, however, believing that just being a "good person" was enough to manage his emotional burdens. This reflects a deeply rooted, though common, stigma around mental health. Some individuals feel that seeking help won't help, is unnecessary, or is a sign of personal weakness or inferiority.

At the age of forty-five, Michael faced a significant health challenge when he was diagnosed with severe Type 2 diabetes. Unfortunately, he never fully acknowledged the reality of his condition, nor did he adhere to proper treatment protocols. This oversight in managing his health led to further complications down the road.

Five years later, at age 50, Michael received a dual diagnosis: Parkinson's disease and early onset dementia. These deteriorating conditions deeply impacted his quality of life. His unresponsiveness and moments of cognitive decline were distressing not only for him but also for his family. He often expressed frustration over his health deterioration, which left him feeling helpless and trapped in a body that was failing him.

As Michael's health continued to decline, his frustration and feelings of abandonment intensified. He faced an overwhelming sense of loss—not just of his physical abilities but also of his identity and role within the family. The combination of chronic illness, emotional burden, and the stigma surrounding mental health likely contributed to his escalating despair.

At the age of 68, a tragic event unfolded. Michael returned to the center field where he had once shone as a Little League star, a place filled with happy memories. In a moment of unbearable pain and hopelessness, he covered himself with a blanket and ended his life with a handgun. This heartbreaking decision shocked and devastated his wife, his children, his 11 grandchildren, and our entire family, leaving a void never be filled.

The medical examiner who completed the autopsy told my sister Mary that her husband's brain was the size and color of a 120-year-old man's.

Michael's life highlights several critical issues surrounding childhood trauma, mental health, chronic illness, and the impact of untreated trauma. Despite being a loving family man, he struggled silently with his internal battles—believing that kindness alone was sufficient for coping without seeking professional assistance. His story serves as a poignant reminder of the importance of addressing childhood trauma and mental health needs, especially when compounded by serious medical conditions.

As we reflect on Michael's life, we remember him as a loving individual whose warmth touched the hearts of many. His tragic end encourages a broader conversation about the significance of mental health support, not just for those who experience trauma directly, but also for their families and communities. It underscores the necessity for empathy, open dialogue, and accessible mental health resources to help prevent such devastating outcomes in the future.

A 2017 meta-analysis of 37 studies, all looking at 23 health outcomes in more than 250,000 people, found the more ACEs a child has, the more likely he or she will have poor health outcomes.[15] Having an ACE score of greater than four increases the probability of diabetes by 52%. The ACEs study reports that having an ACE score greater than six increases the probability of attempting suicide by 950%. Michael's ACE score was seven out of ten.

Let's return to the forest and the topic of Bigfoot.

When you encounter Bigfoot, your amygdala immediately triggers an alarm, signaling your brain to feel fear because Bigfoot is quite frightening! In response, your brain activates both the sympathoadrenal medullary (SAM) and hypothalamic-pituitary-adrenal (HPA) axes, initiating the fight-or-flight response. Signals from the SAM axis travel along nerves from the brain to the adrenal glands, prompting the production of adrenaline, a hormone associated with feelings of terror. Adrenaline causes your heart to beat more forcefully and rapidly, directing blood to essential areas, opening your airways to increase oxygen intake, raising your blood pressure, and redirecting blood flow to your skeletal muscles—critical for running and jumping—while diverting it away from the small muscle that keeps your bladder in check.

Simultaneously, the HPA axis releases hormones in the brain, triggering a cascade of chemical messengers that lead to the production of longer-term stress hormones, particularly cortisol. Imagine living in a forest populated by multiple Bigfoots. After an initial encounter or two, your body would strive to enhance its response to this recurring threat. Essentially, cortisol helps the body adapt to sustained or repeated stressors, such as residing in an environment filled with Bigfoot.

The effects of cortisol mirror those of adrenaline; it elevates blood pressure and blood sugar levels, hinders cognitive function, and destabilizes mood. It also disrupts sleep—an understandable adaptation in a Bigfoot-rich forest, as being a light sleeper could prove beneficial. Unlike adrenaline, which can suppress appetite and stimulate fat burning, cortisol promotes fat accumulation and incites cravings for high-sugar, high-fat foods.

Once you find safety back in your cabin, both the SAM and HPA axes are designed to deactivate. The body employs a mechanism known as feedback inhibition, which prompts the stress response to turn off once its purpose has been fulfilled. Elevated levels of adrenaline and cortisol send signals back to the brain regions responsible for initiating the stress response, effectively shutting them down. It's an impressively evolved system—particularly advantageous for those living in forests prone to Bigfoot. But what happens when safety is elusive? For example, what if Bigfoot returns to your cabin every night?

For Michael, Bigfoot represented his father, who verbally demeaned and physically abused his mother. For Michael and many other survivors, their stress response was activated dozens, if not hundreds, of times each day.

What effects does such relentless adversity have on children's brains and bodies? During my research, I came across compelling work from a 2009 study conducted by researchers Jacqueline Bruce, Phil Fisher, and their colleagues.[16] They aimed to determine whether adverse experiences in preschool-age foster children impacted the functioning of their stress-response system, particularly the HPA axis. This study examined cortisol levels in 117 foster children aged three to six years compared to 60 low-income children who hadn't experienced maltreatment. The researchers found that the foster children showed dysregulated cortisol levels compared to their non-maltreated peers, with different patterns emerging based on the type of trauma. This research provides important evidence of how early adverse experiences affect the functioning of children's stress-response systems, particularly the hypothalamic-pituitary-adrenal (HPA) axis. They discovered that the foster children exhibited dysregulated cortisol levels in contrast to their peers who had not faced similar adversities.

Fisher and Bruce found that children who had experienced maltreatment not only had higher overall cortisol levels but also exhibited a disruption in the normal daily pattern of cortisol secretion.

The key issue is that when the stress response is activated too frequently or when stressors are excessively intense, the body can lose its capacity to shut down the HPA and SAM axes. This phenomenon is referred to as disruption of feedback inhibition, akin to saying that the body's stress thermostat is malfunctioning. Instead of halting the release of "heat" once a certain threshold is reached, it continues to pump cortisol through your system. This is precisely what Fisher and Bruce observed in the foster children.

This persistent hyperactivation of the HPA axis not only affects mental health but also disturbs the delicate balance of other hormones such as insulin, thyroid hormones, and sex hormones, contributing to a host of physiological issues. Prolonged exposure to excessive cortisol can suppress the immune system, elevate blood sugar levels, and even interfere with memory and learning capabilities.

Moreover, childhood trauma can lead to altered functioning of the adrenal glands, which produce hormones essential for maintaining homeostasis. In response to trauma, these glands may become overactive or even exhausted, resulting in a state commonly known as adrenal fatigue. This condition manifests as chronic fatigue, anxiety, and depression, all intertwined with hormonal imbalances. The resulting dysregulation can have far-reaching implications, contributing to metabolic disorders, cardiovascular diseases, and other chronic health conditions.

Research suggests that childhood trauma can also alter the levels and functioning of critical hormones—specifically oxytocin, which plays a key role in social bonding and emotional regulation. These hormonal changes may impair an individual's ability to form healthy relationships and effectively manage emotional responses, further exacerbating the cycle of stress and trauma.

The interplay between childhood trauma and hormonal dysfunction can influence lifestyle choices and behaviors, perpetuating a negative feedback loop. Individuals with a history of trauma may be more prone to engage in maladaptive behaviors such as substance abuse, poor dietary choices, and sedentary lifestyles, which can adversely affect metabolic health and lead to additional hormonal imbalances.

To summarize this crucial point: when a child endures frequent or severe stress, the mechanisms that regulate and deactivate cortisol and adrenaline can malfunction, leading to persistently elevated and unhealthy levels of these hormones throughout adulthood.

Recognizing these connections is crucial for developing effective interventions and support systems aimed at healing and recovery for those affected by childhood trauma.

CHAPTER SIX

Impact of Childhood Trauma on Brain Development

"Research on the effects of early maltreatment tells a different story: that early maltreatment has enduring negative effects on brain development. Our brains are sculpted by our early experiences. Maltreatment is a chisel that shapes a brain to contend with strife, but at the cost of deep, enduring wounds. Childhood abuse isn't something you 'get over.' It is an evil that we must acknowledge and confront if we aim to do anything about the unchecked cycle of violence in this country."

–Martin Teicher, MD, PhD

CHILDHOOD TRAUMA, ENCOMPASSING EXPERIENCES such as abuse, neglect, or severe familial discord, profoundly impacts brain development. In his book *The Body Keeps the Score*, Dr. Bessel van der Kolk reminds us that the actions of those suffering from childhood trauma "are not the result of moral failings or signs of lack of willpower or bad character—they are caused by actual changes in the brain."[17]

The early years of life are critical for shaping neural architecture, as the brain is highly plastic and responsive to environmental stimuli. When a child experiences trauma, the neurodevelopmental process can be significantly altered, leading to long-term consequences.

In normal, healthy brain development, the first few years are characterized by rapid synaptogenesis, where neurons form connections to facilitate learning and social interaction. However, exposure to trauma triggers a stress response, primarily involving the hypothalamic-pituitary-adrenal (HPA) axis. Activation of this stress system results in the release of cortisol and other stress hormones. While short-term stress can enhance certain cognitive functions, chronic exposure to stress-inducing environments disrupts normal brain function, particularly in key regions such as the hippocampus, amygdala, and prefrontal cortex.

The hippocampus, essential for memory formation and emotional regulation, can suffer from reduced volume in children who experience prolonged stress. This shrinkage impacts their ability to learn and process new information, which can manifest as difficulties in academic settings. Similarly, the amygdala, which processes emotions and is instrumental in fear responses, can become hyper-responsive. This hyperactivity may lead to heightened anxiety and hypervigilance, causing children to perceive threats even in safe environments.

The prefrontal cortex, responsible for executive functions such as decision-making, impulse control, and social behavior, often shows delays in maturation due to trauma exposure. Children may find it challenging to regulate their emotions, leading to behavioral issues and difficulty forming stable relationships. These effects can create a cycle of negative reinforcement, where poor emotional regulation leads to further social isolation and potential engagement in risky, even dangerous behaviors.

Dr. Carrion at Stanford University has dedicated significant time to studying children exposed to high levels of adversity. Although prior research in adults indicated that elevated cortisol levels can be harmful to the hippocampus, Dr. Carrion aimed to investigate this phenomenon specifically in children. Utilizing magnetic resonance imaging (MRI) technology, he was able to observe the effects of cortisol on the brains of children who had experienced trauma. What makes Dr. Carrion's work particularly compelling to physicians is that it presents the findings in a framework we are all familiar with. By placing children who had faced adversity into an MRI machine, measurable changes in brain structure became evident.

For this study, Carrion and his team recruited participants from various local health services. The inclusion criteria required the children to have been exposed to trauma, be between the ages of 10 and 16, and exhibit symptoms of PTSD. Most of the children had endured multiple traumatic events, such as witnessing violence or experiencing physical or emotional abuse, and many lived in poverty. The control group consisted of children with no history of trauma, but they were matched to the experimental group in terms of income, age, and race.

During preliminary interviews, researchers asked the children or their caregivers about PTSD symptoms and hyperarousal indicators, including trouble sleeping, irritability, and difficulty concentrating, among others. Each child then underwent an MRI scan, and their salivary cortisol levels were measured four times a day. Once the brain scans were obtained, the researchers assessed the size of each child's hippocampus using 3D volume measurements. They discovered that children with more severe symptoms exhibited higher cortisol levels and smaller hippocampal volumes.

Remarkably, after measuring the hippocampus initially, the researchers conducted follow-up measurements on the same children 12 to 18 months later, revealing that their hippocampi were even smaller. This finding indicated that even though these children were no longer facing trauma, the brain regions responsible for learning and memory continued to shrink, highlighting the lasting impact of earlier stress on their neurological systems.

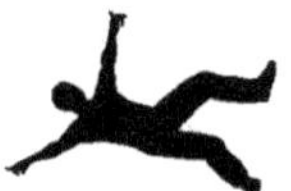

When the amygdala, a key brain region involved in processing fear, is constantly activated by ongoing stress, it becomes overactive. Research using MRI scans has shown that children who suffered severe neglect in Romanian orphanages have altered brain development.[18] This landmark study examined the brain structure of children who had experienced severe early deprivation and found that they had significantly enlarged amygdalae compared to control groups. The researchers also found that these structural differences were associated with difficulties in emotion regulation and anxiety. This is different from the Bruce and Fisher study mentioned earlier, which focused on cortisol levels rather than brain structure. Additionally, when the amygdala is frequently stimulated, it starts to send misleading signals about what is *truly* frightening. This can cause the brain to misidentify threats, leading to unnecessary fear and anxiety.

For children exposed to toxic stress, the activity of the prefrontal cortex, which helps regulate impulses and make thoughtful decisions, is affected in two main ways. First, the overactive amygdala, sensing danger, blunts activity in the prefrontal cortex. Second, the locus coeruleus releases high levels of noradrenaline, which disrupts the brain's ability to manage instincts and impulses. It is as if the brain on high alert is saying, "There's no time to think cooly; do something, and quickly!"

The prefrontal cortex plays a crucial role in helping children control their urges and make safer choices. When a child is told to sit still and concentrate while being bombarded by stress signals, it presents a significant challenge. The resulting impact on the prefrontal cortex varies among individuals. Some may struggle with concentration and problem-solving, while others may exhibit impulsivity and aggression.

This situation raises concerns about the potential for misdiagnosis of attention deficit hyperactivity disorder (ADHD) in students who are actually reacting to extreme stress rather than exhibiting genuine ADHD symptoms.

Case Study 3: Brother Jamie, The Runaway Student

Release a cluster of helium balloons and observe their trajectories. Some will ascend immediately at a rate of eight feet per second, but not all the balloons will rise at the same time. An outlier may bob along the ground, drifting away from the group. Then, for reasons unknown—perhaps an updraft—that outlier suddenly shoots up into the sky, climbing faster and higher than all the others. My brother, Jamie, was that outlier.

The firstborn among 14 siblings, Jamie was—and still is—a larger-than-life figure. He serves as our family's leader, spiritual guide, teacher, and a whirlwind of energy. To know Jamie is to love him.

Much like his father, Jamie embodies an unusual blend of extreme characteristics. Dad taught Jamie from an early age to be a feared street fighter. Jamie was on a path that could easily have led to prison or death. The Jamie we know today is vastly different from the boy described in the early stories within my book, *The Kite That Couldn't Fly*.

Even in grade school, Jamie displayed both gifts and demons. He possessed an undeniable charm that could disarm anyone, yet he also exhibited a rebellious streak and a quick inclination toward physical violence over the slightest provocation. He carried a massive chip on his shoulder. To this day, Jamie remains my protector, but back then, he shared everything he had with me. He was generous and kind, yet also a force of nature. After his First Communion party, he gave me half his gift money, only to put his fist through my first guitar just one day later over a trivial argument.

Jamie had an aversion to school, regularly earning failing grades. In addition to the trauma of neglect and abuse Jamie experienced at home, the nuns at St. Rose grade school also exerted trauma on Jamie in the name of (unsuccessfully) curbing his wildness. Their efforts at physical punishment only strengthened his resolve to disrupt their day. Jamie often strolled off the schoolyard, returning home just in time for dinner. He repeated this routine throughout his grade school years. Mom didn't drive, and Dad was always at work in the factory. Teachers would call Mom, who would then call Dad. Dad would leave work, drive around until he found Jamie, and take him back to school. An hour later, Jamie would walk away again. Eventually, Dad could no longer afford to take time off chasing after Jamie, and as the king of being tough, he reached his breaking point. After one of Dad's searches for him, he warned Jamie that the next time he skipped school, he would receive the beating of his life.

A few days later, Jamie couldn't resist the urge to walk off the playground during morning recess. What puzzled Mom and Dad most about his running away was that Jamie wouldn't engage in any fun or interesting activities once he escaped; he simply wandered around town.

Knowing he was in for hell once Dad found him, Jamie decided to hide well this time. He spotted Dad driving past him several times that day but eventually, Dad gave up. As dusk approached, Jamie's best friend, Tom Dupree, discovered him in one of their familiar hiding spots.

"Jamie, you gotta call your dad. He's sitting at home waiting for you."

Years later, Jamie told me that making that phone call from a payphone was the hardest thing he had ever done. Dad's only reply was, "Where are you? Don't move; I'll be right there."

Sixty years later, while researching for *The Kite That Couldn't Fly*, I was sharing my findings on childhood trauma with Jamie. During one of our almost daily conversations about the book, Jamie revealed that he had been grappling with mild depression, anxiety, and sleeplessness for years. He had sought both medical and mental health assistance, but nothing seemed to help. Diagnosed with ADHD, he took prescribed medication, which brought unwanted side effects and consequences.

Armed with new insights about how childhood trauma can lead to adverse experiences later in life, Jamie began searching for a psychologist who specialized in trauma healing. He found a therapist who listened to his stories about his childhood and adult disorders. The therapist recommended Eye Movement Desensitization and Reprocessing (EMDR) treatment. After just seven sessions Jamie experienced a dramatic reduction in his depression and anxiety and began the process of weaning himself, with his doctor's guidance, off the drugs he was taking for the misdiagnosis of ADHD. Armed with his new awareness, and the aid of EMDR to deal with his fragmented memories, Jamie feels for the first time he is on the path to total healing.

Our adverse childhood experiences are etched into our nervous system and DNA, influencing every aspect of our bodily functions. These factors collectively shape our health, career achievements, relationships, parenting abilities, and even our lifespan due to their profound impact on our bodily systems.

CHAPTER SEVEN

Impact of Childhood Trauma on the Immune System

"The emotional brain controls the production of many chemicals that regulate everything from mood to immune function."

–Dr. Bruce Perry

THE IMMUNE SYSTEM IS our body's defense mechanism, protecting us from harmful pathogens and diseases. Unfortunately, childhood trauma can compromise this system. As we learned, when a child experiences trauma, their body often enters a state of heightened stress response. However, the consequences of toxic stress are not just neurologic and hormonal; they are also immunologic, and those symptoms are much more difficult to spot.

When trauma occurs, the body triggers the fight-or-flight response (like escaping from that Bigfoot), releasing stress hormones such as cortisol and adrenaline. While these hormones are essential for immediate survival, prolonged exposure—often a result of ongoing trauma—can lead to harmful effects. Chronic stress from such trauma can lead to elevated cortisol levels, which, if sustained, can disrupt the balance of the immune system, thus putting the body at greater risk of infection and illness.

Persistent high levels of cortisol can lead to a decrease in the production of immune cells, which are essential for fighting infections. These immune cells, like lymphocytes and macrophages, play key roles in recognizing and eliminating pathogens. Without sufficient levels of these cells, a child's ability to fend off illnesses is compromised. As a result, children who have experienced trauma may find themselves getting sick more frequently or struggling to recover from illnesses.

Moreover, trauma can also exacerbate inflammation in the body. When the immune system is activated repeatedly due to stress, the body may produce inflammatory substances that can lead to chronic inflammation. This condition can increase the risk of developing autoimmune disorders, allergies, and other chronic health problems, further complicating a child's overall well-being.

Researchers in Dunedin, New Zealand, demonstrated that changes in inflammation levels can be quantitatively measured.[19] Over a span of 30 years, they followed a group of 1,000 individuals, meticulously observing and recording a variety of significant health data. In addition to corroborating the findings of Drs. Felitti and Anda, the Dunedin researchers discovered that even 20 years after experiencing childhood maltreatment, participants exhibited elevated levels of four distinct markers of inflammation compared to those who had not experienced maltreatment. The more inflammation there is in the body, the greater the chance that some of that inflammation will attack the body's own tissues, leading to autoimmune diseases like rheumatoid arthritis, inflammatory bowel disease, and multiple sclerosis.

This study is a crucial contribution to the research on Adverse Childhood Experiences (ACEs) because the participants' reports of adverse events were documented as they occurred. This strengthens the argument for causality by establishing that the adversity preceded the patient's biological effects.

Understanding this physical connection is crucial for caregivers, educators, and health professionals who can provide better support to children facing such challenges, helping them build resilience and improve their health. Better support is also required for the adults whose trauma has manifested into mental and physical disorders and illnesses. Healthcare professionals need to shift from treating mere symptoms to digging into the root causes, and when appropriate, recommending trauma counseling.

Did our childhood adversity threaten our immune system as much as it did our mental well-being? The problem was that, for us, no one suspected that our immune system could be compromised by toxic stress.

No one knew where to look.

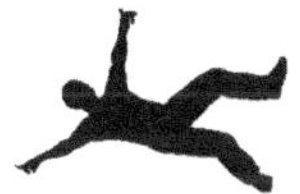

Case Study 4: The Impact of Childhood Trauma on Immune Function
A Personal Investigation

Background

Childhood is a critical period for physical, emotional, and sensory development. Psychological trauma, particularly stemming from poverty and neglect, may have long-lasting effects on an individual's health, including their immune system. This case study aims to explore the potential connections between childhood trauma and compromised immune function, using the experiences of two siblings—myself and my brother, Allen—as prominent examples.

Subject Profiles

1. Subject A (Self)

- Age: 75

- Health History:

  ○ Frequent illnesses in childhood, primarily colds that developed into strep throat.

  ○ Lack of access to medical care due to poverty, resulting in untreated health issues.

  ○ At age sixteen, developed Rheumatic Fever necessitating a six-month hospital stay. The illness attacked the heart and damaged the aortic valve.

  ○ History of an infected aortic valve leading to open-heart surgery at age sixty-nine.

  ○ Suffered a stroke two weeks post-surgery, followed by a serious chest infection requiring extensive antibiotic treatment, which resulted in dual foot neuropathy.

As a child, recurrent strep throat and frequent colds were indicative of a compromised immune system. The escalation to Rheumatic Fever indicates an immune response heavily influenced by early neglect and lack of preventive care. The resulting cardiac issues highlight how early trauma potentially contributed to chronic health problems in adulthood.

2. Subject B (Allen)
- Age at Death: 46

- Health History:

  - Lack of access to medical care due to poverty, resulting in poorly treated health issues.

  - Similar pattern of frequent illnesses, including recurrent pneumonia leading to hospitalization.

  - Passed away from colon cancer, raising questions about chronic immune system and health compromise.

Allen's hospitalizations for pneumonia in childhood suggest a similar pattern of immune dysfunction. His untimely death from colon cancer raises further questions about the long-term effects of childhood illness and trauma on overall health and cancer susceptibility.

Both subjects grew up in a lower socioeconomic environment characterized by limited access to healthcare, food insecurity, and emotional neglect. This environment not only affected physical health but also placed them at greater risk for developing long-term health complications. The absence of medical care during crucial developmental years might have hindered their immune system maturation, leading to increased susceptibility to infections and serious illness.

In van der Kolk's book, *The Body Keeps the Score*, he makes the compelling case that childhood adversity can lead to dysregulation of the immune system, increased inflammation, and a higher likelihood of chronic diseases later in life. The combined health issues of the pair of siblings suggest a possible correlation between the childhood trauma they experienced and their immune system's effectiveness in combating infections. Consider the following:

1. **Psychological and Physical Stress:** Childhood trauma can trigger chronic stress responses that may alter immune function and overall health. The biological impacts of stress hormones, such as cortisol, can impair the immune response, leaving individuals vulnerable to infections and diseases.
2. **Social Determinants of Health:** Growing up in poverty typically correlates with inadequate healthcare access, nutrition, and stability, all critical components of a healthy immune system. The social context likely compounded the siblings' vulnerabilities.
3. **Long-term Health Consequences:** The lack of early medical intervention and treatment for recurrent health issues may have established a pattern of chronic illness, reinforcing the idea that early trauma and neglect can lead to adverse health outcomes.

Conclusion

While it is difficult to definitively establish a causal relationship, the shared health challenges of myself and my brother Allen prompt an essential examination of childhood trauma's lasting impact on immune function and overall well-being. We could all benefit from future research that explores the mechanisms through which socioeconomic factors and emotional neglect contribute to long-term health disparities. Understanding these links may offer deeper insights into preventive healthcare and strategies to mitigate the effects of childhood adversity on health.

I want to clarify that I do not share these stories to seek sympathy or pity, nor do I wish to assign blame to my parents for the neglect we experienced during our childhood. I genuinely believe they did the best they could with the resources and circumstances available to them. My intention in sharing these personal experiences is to highlight the profound impact that a compromised immune system can have later in life, illustrating how early adversity can manifest in significant health challenges as we grow older.

As we have explored, childhood trauma can profoundly affect a child's development, leading to disruptions in physical health, emotional well-being, and social functioning. The stress response affects our hormones, brain function, and immune system, making it the biggest indicator of the lasting effects of the trauma itself. This means, the aftermath of ACEs forms a crucial aspect of understanding not only individual lives but the broader implications for society as these children grow into adults carrying the burdens of their past.

Chapter Eight

Destruction & Disintegration

"Childhood trauma plants the seeds of despair; if left unaddressed, they can grow into a forest of pain and disintegration."

–Unknown

As I write this chapter, I experience a sensation that transcends writer's block; it feels more like a paralyzing sadness, a weight that threatens to smother my motivation and commitment to write this book. How does one even begin to articulate the breadth and depth of destruction wrought by experiences that began in such innocent moments?

The body of evidence I've amassed is staggering, revealing an unsettling truth about the impact of childhood trauma. Each time I dive into my research notes, I find myself confronting statistics from studies and personal conversations that feel almost unbelievable—so profound that they leave me momentarily lost in despair over the magnitude of suffering they represent. This overwhelming realization leads me to procrastinate, at times tempting me to set aside this project altogether. Sometimes, the problem feels too insurmountable to tackle. Yet, in those moments of uncertainty, a powerful quote by Elie Wiesel echoes in my mind.

"We are each responsible for the evil we do not prevent."

This thought becomes my anchor, compelling me to push through the discomfort and resume this crucial work. The voice within reminds me that I somehow have a responsibility to illuminate these issues, no matter how daunting the task may seem.

Before we continue, I want to make clear what I mean by "disintegration." This refers to the process of breaking down or the loss of cohesion and integrity within an individual's mental, physical, spiritual, and social dimensions. In the aftermath of childhood trauma, disintegration manifests as fragmented thoughts, emotions, and behaviors that disrupt a person's sense of self and connection to the world around them. This deterioration can lead to symptoms such as emotional numbness, physical ailments, spiritual disconnection, and interpersonal difficulties.

It's also important to establish a foundation of understanding regarding causality. Causation, in this context, refers to the relationship between childhood trauma and the various psychological and physical disorders that emerge later in life. This is not a mere correlation; rather, research—including the pivotal findings of the ACEs study—that demonstrates a direct link between early exposure to trauma and the development of these conditions.

While I recognize I may not capture every disorder or dysfunctional behavior that can be traced back to childhood trauma, the wealth of data available to us today provides a strong basis for asserting these causal connections. We stand on the shoulders of countless researchers who have dedicated their lives to uncovering these truths, enabling us to speak with confidence and conviction about the lingering shadows cast by childhood trauma.

In grappling with the almost unbelievable, yet painfully real, consequences of childhood trauma, my conviction and authority are deeply rooted in my own lived experience. Growing up in a family of fourteen siblings, I have witnessed and endured a wide spectrum of childhood neglect, abuse, and familial dysfunction. This heartbreaking reality has manifested in an array of outcomes for my siblings and me, spanning from mild depression and anxiety to the extreme tragedy of suicide. Our experiences have not only shaped our emotional landscapes but have also given rise to numerous disorders and health issues, including obesity, diabetes, heart disease, alcoholism, drug addiction, teen pregnancies, incarceration, and the worst of all disintegration, premature death.

As it turns out, my family is a microcosm of humanity; a metaphorical petri dish you can look at under a microscope. This serves as a stark reminder of the pervasive and very real impact of childhood adversities, allowing me to write with a depth of understanding and passion that transcends statistics. I intend to illustrate just how profoundly and multifacetedly childhood trauma can ripple across generations.

It is time to confront the harsh realities that manifest from childhood trauma—an experience that cannot only create pain and unhappiness to the child, but also trigger an array of disorders, illnesses, and profound deterioration across physical, mental, social, and spiritual dimensions.

As we've already learned, the impact of trauma is far-reaching, often leaving scars that extend well beyond childhood and into adulthood. Further, it is one of the most insidious and contagious afflictions in our world today.

As you continue to read this book, I encourage you to maintain that sense of alarm and concern. Use it as a lens through which to examine the pervasive impacts of childhood trauma in our world today. To date the statistics have not made headlines, but they reveal a very real, silent epidemic that demands our collective awareness and action.

I want to clarify that I'm not encouraging a relentless search for hidden trauma; not every struggle we face in adulthood can be traced back to childhood experiences. Disorders and illnesses have various origins, and many factors contribute to their development. Nevertheless, given that approximately 70% of all adults in the US report having experienced some form of childhood trauma, it is worth considering the potential connections between early experiences and present-day challenges. Recognizing this link can promote understanding and healing, but it is crucial to do so without placing undue blame on past events or triggering unnecessary anxiety about memories that may never surface.

The outcomes of childhood trauma are undeniably tragic, and while each disorder and dysfunction deserve acknowledgment, I will begin with the most distressing manifestations—those that lead to a sense of surrender. Many individuals find themselves losing hope, becoming numb to the world around them, and in some cases, they are tragically propelled into homelessness. These people have withdrawn from the pursuit of healing and redemption, feeling trapped in an existence devoid of possibility.

Understanding this landscape of destruction is crucial. This awareness opens the door to compassion, urging us to not only acknowledge these profound effects but to seek pathways for healing and restoration, both for individuals and for society as a whole.

Let's begin with Camilla's story.

Case Study 5: Camilla's Story Heavy Burden

Camilla, a 50-year-old woman, lives a life shadowed by the weight of her past and the complexities of her present. The journey of her existence has been marred by a series of traumatic experiences that not only altered the course of her life but also left deep emotional and physical scars. After reading my book, *The Kite That Couldn't Fly*, she reached out to me in a moment of desperation, drawn by a glimmer of hope that perhaps sharing her story with someone could provide hope for healing.

Her voice trembled as she spoke, revealing the pain beneath each word, crafted by the haunting echoes of a challenging childhood. With an Adverse Childhood Experiences (ACEs) score of 10, Camilla's early life was a mosaic of neglect, abuse, and instability. The impact of these experiences manifested into a complex landscape of mental health struggles; she was diagnosed with four different mental illnesses—depression, anxiety, bipolar and schizophrenia—a testament to the depth of her emotional pain. Further, her daily existence is overshadowed by a myriad of physical health issues, including diabetes, obesity, and cardiac disease, which serve as constant reminders of her plight.

Camilla's connection with her family has disintegrated, leaving her isolated and vulnerable. The dissolution of her marriage and the subsequent estrangement from her children deepen her sense of despair. The family bonds that should provide comfort are now a source of heartache, pushing her further into the abyss. She lost her job and struggles to make ends meet. Each day becomes a battle, marked by an overwhelming sense of paralysis that grips her limbs and mind alike. She told me that getting out of bed can feel like a Herculean task; the floor beneath her seems to conspire against her efforts, enforcing a gravitational weight that both physically and metaphorically pulls her down. In her mind, this sensation embodies the emotional turmoil and persistent struggle that have defined her existence.

Maybe the worst of Camilla's symptoms was her emotional numbness. She desperately wanted to love her family, but she couldn't seem to feel any deep connection to them. Camilla felt emotionally distant from everyone, as though her heart were frozen, and she were living behind a glass wall. This numbness also extended to her own sense of self; she struggled to feel anything beyond brief flashes of anger and overwhelming shame. When she looked in the mirror, she hardly recognized the person staring back at her.

After divulging her struggles to me, she whispered weakly, "It's a force so strong I can hardly move."

In sharing her story, Camilla opened my eyes to the lived reality of many who suffer in silence. Her day-to-day existence is fraught with the contemplation of suicide, a stark acknowledgment of her darkest thoughts. Yet, in the brief interlude of our conversation, Camilla revealed a flicker of hope—her desire to break free from the cycle of suffering, to find a reason to rise above the confines of her mind and body. She said my story was one of beautiful redemption. She longs for connection, for understanding, and for a way to transform her narrative into one of resilience rather than despair.

I listened to her with a lump in my throat. Camilla's story serves as a poignant reminder of the profound effects of childhood trauma and the ripple effects that continue throughout one's life. I wonder if this is how my brothers Patrick and Adam felt before they died from drug overdoses.

Camilla's story is a call to action for society to recognize and address the silent struggles of those who have endured their own kites failing to fly. While her journey is fraught with obstacles, it is also filled with potential for healing. The path ahead may be tumultuous, but with support, understanding, and a willingness to confront the past, it is possible for Camilla—and many like her—to discover a newfound strength and reclaim their stories. In our shared conversation, I realized that sometimes it takes a single voice to advocate for change and resilience, and Camilla's deserves to be heard.

After listening intently, I gave Camilla my rehearsed response. "I am so sorry for your pain, for what you have experienced and are experiencing now. I know you are calling with hope that I might be able to help you. You need to know I am not a doctor or a metal health professional. But I can tell you what you are experiencing does not need to be a life sentence." I told her that the book by Dr. Glenn Schiraldi, *The Adverse Childhood Experiences Workbook,* was a Godsend for me. I gave her a suicide prevention phone number and asked her to use it anytime she felt at risk of taking her life.

Camilla believes her feeling of being pulled down to the ground is due to her depression and other mental illnesses. While some of the symptoms of depression fall neatly into the category of mental illness, we are now learning that such sensations and feeling might be due to malfunctioning metabolism. In his groundbreaking book, *Brain Energy*, Dr. Christopher Palmer explains that changes in sleep, energy, motivation, and concentration likely all relate to reduced function of brain cells.[20] The fatigue almost certainly extends to the muscles throughout the body, given that mitochondrial dysfunction has been found there, too.

In some cases, people will describe "leaden paralysis," a situation in which they feel like their arms and legs are made of lead and it's difficult to even move them. This is exactly how Camilla described feeling when she attempts to get out of bed. Mitochondrial dysfunction in her muscles might explain this. If her muscles don't have enough energy, she will have difficulty moving them. Catatonia is a complex syndrome, most seen in people with underlying mood or psychotic disorders. It's an extreme version of metabolic failure—people can appear paralyzed from their illness and have severe difficulty moving or speaking.

For Camilla, the struggle she faces may not solely be a matter of willpower or mental fortitude; it could also reflect deeper, biological challenges that require comprehensive attention. By acknowledging this connection, we can better understand the multifaceted nature of her experience, paving the way for a more holistic approach to healing that encompasses both mental and physical health. Understanding the interplay between these elements may ultimately provide Camilla—and others like her—with a clearer pathway towards recovery and a renewed sense of hope.

Research has indicated that trauma can lead to long-term alterations in bodily systems, including hormonal and metabolic pathways. These changes can manifest as fatigue, depression, and pervasive low energy, making even the simplest tasks, like getting out of bed, feel insurmountable. It is essential to recognize that trauma doesn't just reside in the mind; it can ripple through our entire physiology, impacting everything from brain chemistry to metabolic function.

So many people suffer greatly long past the initial traumatic experience. They stay stagnant in pain and loss, unable to recover or even return to some semblance of life before trauma. They're paralyzed by all they've lost and by the pain they continue to feel. They may feel overwhelmed and without the hope or resources to recover.

CHAPTER NINE

Quantifying the Destruction

"The scale of the trauma in our country is almost unfathomable. We've become so accustomed to the casualties that we don't even see them anymore."
–Dr. Nadine Burke Harris, California's First Surgeon General

THROUGHOUT THIS BOOK, YOU will witness the unbelievable amount of destruction and disintegration childhood trauma creates across four dimensions: physical, mental, social, and spiritual. The evidence is overwhelming, the research irrefutable, and the personal stories heartbreaking. But perhaps nothing drives home the true scope of this crisis like the raw numbers—the cold, hard mathematics of how childhood trauma is systematically destroying American society.

This chapter quantifies the destruction across four critical areas that demonstrate just how powerfully childhood trauma is pulling down our society:

- How it has become the leading cause of death in America while we've been counting the bodies all wrong;

- How it drives the vast majority of addiction and substance abuse;

- How it is the primary engine behind our suicide epidemic; and

- How it fills our prisons through a predictable pathway from childhood trauma to adult incarceration.

Finally, we'll confront the millions of walking wounded—the "unseen" army of survivors moving through our communities, carrying invisible wounds that bleed in public spaces while the world looks away.

These numbers aren't just statistics—they represent hundreds of thousands of preventable deaths, millions of destroyed lives, and trillions of dollars in societal costs. More importantly, they reveal the true enemy we're fighting: not individual moral failures or character flaws, but a systematic pattern of childhood trauma that has infected our society like a virus, spreading from generation to generation with precision.

The Hidden Death Toll: America's #1 Killer

For decades, we've been looking at the aftermath of childhood trauma without seeing the source. We count heart disease deaths, cancer deaths, overdoses, and suicides as separate issues, but never connect them to their common root. When we follow the data, we uncover the lethal toll that changes everything we thought we knew about mortality in America: Severe childhood trauma is killing 1,401 Americans every single day, making it the leading cause of death in our nation.[21]

Read that again. Not the third-leading cause. Not the second. The *leading* cause of death in the United States of America.

To understand how we missed this, you need to know how we've been counting wrong.

We've Been Counting the Bodies All Wrong

Death certificates record what people die *from*—the final medical event. They don't record what people die *because of*—the root cause that set the disease process in motion decades earlier.

When a 52-year-old man dies of a heart attack, his death certificate reads "heart disease." When a 34-year-old woman dies of a drug overdose, it reports "accidental poisoning." When a 19-year-old takes his own life, it says "suicide." When a 3-year-old is beaten to death, it's named "homicide."

But what if all four deaths shared the same root cause? What if decades of peer-reviewed research proved that a single, preventable factor was driving all of them?

That factor is childhood trauma.

The 33.2 million Americans with ACE scores of 4 or higher—those who experienced the most severe childhood trauma—die an average of 20 years earlier than those who don't.[22] When these people die of heart disease at 55 instead of 75, the death certificate reads "myocardial infarction." When they overdose at 30, it's labeled "accidental poisoning." When they take their own life at 25, it's deemed "suicide." But strip away the medical terminology, and you see the truth: Trauma is the cause and these are its symptoms.

The Mathematics of Misattribution

Current death certificate methodology fundamentally miscounts mortality by recording only the final medical event rather than the root cause. The biological pathway from trauma to death is scientifically established:

Childhood Trauma → Toxic Stress → Neurobiological Changes → Behavioral Adaptations → Disease → Death

Using Population Attributable Fraction (PAF) methodology—the same approach that proved smoking causes lung cancer—researchers have now calculated what percentage of deaths from various causes would be prevented if childhood trauma were eliminated.[21]

The landmark Grummitt study, published in *JAMA* Pediatrics in December 2021, analyzed data from over 20 million participants across 19 meta-analyses. The researchers—from Harvard, Columbia, and the University of Sydney—found that childhood adversity is directly attributable to 439,072 U.S. deaths per year. But critically, their study *excluded drug overdose deaths* because insufficient meta-analyses existed at the time.[21]

That was a massive gap. With over 105,000 overdose deaths per year[1] and 67% or more attributable to childhood trauma,[23, 24] the true death toll was understated by approximately 70,000 deaths annually.

When you add the drug overdose deaths back in, plus direct child deaths from abuse and neglect, the total reaches 511,427 deaths per year—making childhood trauma the number one cause of death in America.

Cause of Death	Annual Deaths	Deaths Per Day
Heart Disease	219,470	601
Cancer	82,888	227
Drug Overdose	70,355	193
Chronic Lower Respiratory Disease	66,702	183
Suicide	39,686	109
Stroke	26,758	73
Diabetes	3,568	10
Child Abuse/Neglect Fatalities	2,000	5
TOTAL	**511,427**	**1,401**

Annual Deaths Attributable to Childhood Trauma

A note on child fatalities: The 2,000 children killed each year by abuse and neglect represent the most immediate and tragic deaths from childhood trauma. These children never had the chance to develop heart disease or cancer—they were killed before they could grow up. Federal data indicates that 50-60% of child maltreatment fatalities are not recorded on death certificates as such, meaning the true number is likely higher.[25]

The Daily Death Toll

The 511,427 annual deaths attributable to childhood trauma translates to 1,401 deaths per day. One death every 61 seconds. 58 deaths per hour. Nearly six children and 1,395 adults die daily from the consequences of childhood trauma—either immediately or decades later when their bodies can no longer bear the biological burden of their earliest experiences.

Let those numbers sink in. While you read this chapter, approximately 20 Americans will die from the long-term effects of childhood trauma. By the time you finish this book, thousands more will be gone.

Leading Root Causes of Death in America

Death certificates record mechanisms of death—heart attack, cancer, overdose. To understand what's actually killing Americans, we must identify root causes: the upstream factors that trigger these diseases years or decades before death.[26]

Unlike death certificate categories like heart disease and cancer, root causes can be *prevented*. When compared to other preventable root causes, childhood trauma is number one.[1,21,27,28,29]

For decades, tobacco held that grim distinction. We spent billions on anti-smoking campaigns, passed laws restricting cigarette advertising, required warning labels, banned smoking in public places. And it worked—smoking rates dropped from 42% of American adults in 1965 to about 11% today.

These are all root causes—upstream factors that trigger disease and death:

Rank	Root Cause of Death	Annual Deaths
#1	Childhood Trauma	511,427
#2	Tobacco	480,000
#3	Poor Diet / Physical Inactivity	~300,000
#4	Alcohol (excessive use)	178,000
#5	Microbial Agents (infections)	~75,000
#6	Toxic Agents (pollutants, asbestos)	~55,000
#7	Motor Vehicle Crashes	~43,000
#8	Firearms	~43,000

Leading Root Causes of Death in America

Childhood trauma has been quietly killing more Americans than tobacco ever did. And we've done almost nothing about it.

Why Has No One Discovered This Before?

If childhood trauma truly is the leading cause of death in America, why hasn't the medical establishment—the CDC, or any major researcher—identified this before? The answer lies in seven structural barriers that have kept this truth hidden:

1. **Death Certificates Don't Record Root Causes.** The entire mortality reporting system is designed to capture the final medical event, not what caused it. A coroner writes "myocardial infarction," not "childhood abuse triggered chronic inflammation that destroyed this

person's cardiovascular system over 40 years." The system literally cannot see root causes.

2. **The ACEs Research Is Relatively New.** The landmark CDC-Kaiser ACE Study wasn't published until 1998. The scientific understanding of how childhood trauma causes adult disease is barely 25 years old.

3. **The PAF Mortality Data Only Became Available in 2021.** The Grummitt study—the first to calculate Population Attributable Fraction for childhood trauma across multiple disease categories—wasn't published until December 2021.[21] Before that, researchers knew childhood trauma increased disease risk, but no one had calculated how many actual deaths it caused.

4. **Drug Overdose Deaths Were Excluded.** Even the groundbreaking Grummitt study explicitly excluded drug overdose deaths because insufficient meta-analyses existed at the time. With 105,000 overdose deaths per year[1] and 67% or more attributable to ACEs,[23,24] this was a massive gap that understated the true death toll by approximately 70,000 deaths annually.

5. **Medical Specialization Creates Silos.** Cardiologists study hearts. Oncologists study cancer. Addiction specialists study substance use. Pediatricians see children. No one is incentivized to connect the dots across all these specialties to see that childhood trauma is driving disease in ALL of them.

6. **The Deaths Are Spread Across Decades.** When someone is abused at age five and dies of a heart attack at age 55, the connection isn't obvious. Fifty years separate cause from effect. Unlike immediate causes like a car accident killing its driver, the delayed mortality effect of childhood trauma requires sophisticated epidemiological analysis to detect.

7. **No Economic or Political Incentive to Connect the Dots.** There's a powerful pharmaceutical industry selling heart medications, cancer

treatments, and addiction drugs. There's no equivalent "childhood trauma prevention" industry lobbying for recognition. No one profits from preventing the disease before it starts.

The Discovery Required an Outsider's Perspective

Sometimes it takes someone outside the medical establishment—someone trained to see systems, connect data across domains, and challenge fundamental assumptions—to see what specialists cannot.

As an inventor with 14 patents who has advised NASA and the United Nations on complex systems problems, I approached this question the way I approach any engineering challenge: follow the data, ignore conventional categories, and don't stop until you find root cause. Engineers don't accept "it's complicated" as an answer. We dig until we find the single point of failure that's bringing down the whole system.

When I began researching childhood trauma after writing my memoir *The Kite That Couldn't Fly*, I wasn't constrained by academic silos. I didn't see cardiology and oncology and addiction medicine as separate fields. I saw inputs and outputs. Causes and effects. A system with a massive failure rate—and a root cause that everyone was ignoring.

The data was there. The Grummitt study was published. The PAF research on addiction was available. The CDC child fatality statistics were public. Someone just needed to put the pieces together.

I put the pieces together. And when I did, I realized we've been counting the bodies all wrong.

The Addiction Engine: How Trauma Creates Its Own Medicine

The connection between childhood trauma and addiction isn't correlation—it's causation with a clear biological pathway. When children experience trauma, their developing brains are flooded with stress hormones that damage the very structures responsible for emotional regulation, impulse control, and stress management. These damaged brains then desperately seek external chemicals to restore what trauma destroyed internally.

The Statistical Proof

The numbers are staggering. Research shows that 67-72% of all substance use disorders are directly attributable to Adverse Childhood Experiences.[23,24] The relationship follows a clear dose-response pattern: more trauma equals higher addiction risk.

- 1-2 ACEs: 2x increased risk of drug use

- 3-4 ACEs: 5x increased risk

- 5+ ACEs: 7-10x increased risk

- 6+ ACEs: 4,600% increased risk of injection drug use[30]

Adults with any history of ACEs have a 5.3-fold higher likelihood of developing substance use disorders, with females showing a 5.9-fold increase for alcohol disorders and males showing a 5.0-fold increase for illicit drug disorders.[31]

The Fentanyl Crisis Is Actually a Trauma Crisis

We're told America has a "fentanyl crisis" or an "opioid epidemic." But fentanyl didn't create addicts—it killed people who were already addicted. And what made them addicts?

The research is unequivocal: 67-72% of addiction can be traced to childhood trauma.[23,24] An estimated 70-80% of adolescent opioid misuse is attributable to ACEs.[23]

People don't become addicted because drugs feel good. They become addicted because childhood pain feels unbearable.[32] Drugs provide temporary relief from chronic toxic stress embedded in their bodies from early adversity.

Why Substances "Work"

Traumatized individuals don't randomly choose substances—they unconsciously select drugs that temporarily correct their specific neurobiological deficits:

- **Opioids** replace depleted endorphins and provide the warmth absent in childhood

- **Stimulants** compensate for prefrontal cortex damage from trauma

- **Alcohol** reduces amygdala hyperactivity and temporarily decreases anxiety

- **Cannabis** regulates the disrupted endocannabinoid system

The cruel irony: Substances that initially correct trauma-induced deficits ultimately worsen them. Tolerance develops, withdrawal recreates original trauma symptoms, and the brain adapts by deepening dysfunction. The "solution" becomes the problem.

The Biological Murder: When Childhood Trauma Becomes Suicide

Michael Kohl died by suicide at age 68. During the autopsy, the coroner discovered something that should shake the foundation of how we understand suicide: his brain had the size and color of a 120-year-old man's brain. The cause wasn't age—it was childhood trauma.

Michael's ACE score was 7. For 11 years, he watched his alcoholic father beat his mother. For 11 years, his developing brain was flooded with cortisol. For 11 years, his mitochondria were systematically destroyed. The trauma didn't end when the beatings stopped—it continued its silent destruction for another 54 years, until his brain could no longer sustain life.

The Evidence

The evidence that childhood trauma is the primary cause of suicide is overwhelming:

- **89.4% of suicide attempts** among high school students are attributable to ACEs[33]

- **80% of adult suicide deaths** are conservatively attributable to childhood trauma[21]

- Adults with 4+ ACEs face a **51-fold increased risk** of suicide attempts[34]

In 2023, 49,449 Americans died by suicide. Based on population attributable fraction data, 39,686 of these deaths (80%) were attributable to childhood trauma.[21] That's 109 people per day—4.5 people per hour—dying by suicide from the long-term effects of ACEs.

The Neurobiological Pathway to Death

Michael Kohl's brain tells the story of trauma's lethality. Childhood trauma triggers a biological cascade:

1. Trauma activates the stress response system, flooding the brain with cortisol

2. Chronic cortisol exposure directly damages mitochondria—the cellular powerhouses

3. Brain cells begin dying from energy starvation

4. Critical brain regions shrink and lose function

5. Accelerated aging occurs at the cellular level

6. The brain literally ages faster than chronological time

Michael's autopsy revealed a brain with 20% below normal weight, gray-brown color instead of healthy pink, severely atrophied hippocampus, and mitochondrial density 60% below normal.[35] This is what childhood trauma looks like at autopsy—a brain destroyed by decades of biological damage initiated in childhood.

Suicide Is Not a Choice

The evidence forces us to confront reality: suicide is not weakness, selfishness, or moral failing. It is the endpoint of neurobiological destruction—the result of cellular death, the consequence of mitochondrial failure, the culmination of decades of damage. Michael Kohl didn't choose to die. His brain, destroyed by 60 years of trauma-initiated degeneration, could no longer sustain life.

From Cradle to Cage: How Incarceration Manufactures Itself

The United States has constructed the most efficient self-perpetuating system of human suffering in modern history. We call it criminal justice, but it is a machine that creates its own fuel—a cycle so perfectly designed to perpetuate itself through childhood trauma that it appears almost intentional.

The Numbers Don't Lie

The disparity between general and incarcerated populations reveals trauma's dominance:

- **98% of prisoners** have at least one ACE (vs. 64% general population)

- **45–46% of prisoners** have 4+ ACEs (vs. 17% general population)

- **Avg. ACE score of prisoners:** 5.0 (vs. 1.6 general population)[32]

Intergenerational Amplification

Here's where the system becomes truly insidious. Parental incarceration is itself an ACE, affecting 2.7 million American children. Among incarcerated populations:

- **45% of men** had a family member incarcerated during childhood (vs. 9% general population)

- **40% of women** had family incarceration during childhood (vs. 8% general population)[37]

Children with incarcerated parents face:
- 6x higher risk of juvenile incarceration

- 5x higher risk of adult incarceration

- 3x higher risk of behavioral problems

- 2x higher risk of mental health disorders[38]

The Perfect Circle of Suffering

The cycle is precise:

Childhood Trauma (ACEs) → Neurobiological Changes → Behavioral Adaptations → Criminalization of Trauma Responses → Incarceration → Creates Childhood Trauma in Next Generation → Cycle Repeats Infinitely

This isn't a flaw in the system—this *is* the system. Each generation doesn't just inherit trauma—it compounds it. We are literally traumatizing children and creating prisoners.

The Unseen: Trauma's Shadow Army

They walk among us every day—millions of souls carrying invisible wounds that bleed in public spaces while the world looks away. In back alleys, behind prison walls, in psychiatric wards, and in the darkest corners of our cities, childhood trauma has created an army of the unseen.

The Faces of Hidden Trauma

The homeless man wrapped in a tattered blanket didn't choose the streets—the streets chose him when he was eight and his stepfather's fists taught him that home was the most dangerous place on earth. His brain, desperate to survive, learned that sleeping outdoors felt safer than sleeping indoors. Forty years later, he still can't close his eyes in enclosed spaces without his nervous system screaming danger.

The woman selling her body on a dark corner wasn't born for this life—she was groomed for it by the uncle who "loved" her when she was 12. Her brain, rewiring itself around betrayal and violation, learned that her body was currency before she learned multiplication tables.

The man behind bars didn't wake up one day and choose violence—violence chose him before he could walk, when his mother's boyfriend decided a crying baby needed to be silenced with shaken bones and bruised skin. His developing brain adapted to chaos, learning that striking first meant surviving another day.

The Mathematics of the Unseen

Behind every statistic is a story that began in childhood:

- 2.5 million Americans experience homelessness each year, most carrying trauma from before they learned to tie their shoes

- 1 million people trapped in sex trafficking, their nervous systems conditioned by childhood abuse to accept exploitation as normal

- 21 million Americans struggling with addiction, their pain so deep that poisoning themselves feels like relief

- 7 million adults with severe mental illness, their minds shattered by betrayals that happened before they knew what betrayal meant[39]

Invisible Chains

What the world sees as moral failure, science reveals as neurobiological adaptation. What society labels as choice, research exposes as consequence. The homeless man's inability to maintain housing isn't laziness—it's a nervous system that equates enclosed spaces with terror. The sex worker's return to the streets isn't moral deficiency—it's a brain that learned to associate love with exploitation. The prisoner's violence isn't evil—it's a fight-or-flight response that he never learned to turn off.

The Children They Once Were

Before they became the unseen, they were children with dreams. The homeless man once built elaborate forts and dreamed of becoming an architect. The sex worker once danced in her bedroom mirror, pretending to be a ballerina. The prisoner once collected bugs and dreamed of becoming a scientist. Trauma didn't erase those dreams—it buried them under survival strategies that made tomorrow possible but joy impossible.

The Ultimate Reckoning

When you add it all up—the 511,427 annual deaths, the 21 million Americans struggling with addiction, the 49,449 suicides, the 2 million incarcerated individuals, the millions of unseen walking wounded—you realize we're not just facing a public health crisis. We're witnessing the slow-motion collapse of human potential on a scale that dwarfs every other challenge we face.

Climate change gets headlines. The economy gets congressional hearings. Meanwhile, childhood trauma quietly destroys more lives than cancer, claims more victims than accidents, and costs more than our entire defense budget. The annual economic burden of ACEs is estimated at $748 billion in North America alone—more than the GDP of most nations.[40]

The Mirror We Must Face

The unseen force us to confront uncomfortable truths: We are only a few traumatic experiences away from joining their ranks; our housed, employed, functional lives exist partly because we were lucky enough to avoid the worst childhood experiences; their visible pain reflects invisible wounds carried by millions more who have learned to hide their bleeding.

Every unseen person represents a cascade of lost potential. The homeless man who might have designed buildings that housed thousands instead lies under bridges. The sex worker who might have danced on Broadway instead performs for survival on street corners. The prisoner who might have discovered cures for diseases instead is locked away from the world he could have healed.

The Choice Before Us

We can continue to criminalize trauma responses, or we can finally address childhood trauma itself. We can keep building more prisons, shelters, and psychiatric wards, or we can start building trauma-responsive communities that prevent these casualties in the first place. We can keep averting our eyes from the unseen, or we can finally see them as the wounded children they still are inside broken adult bodies.

The data conclusively demonstrates that childhood trauma constitutes the *leading* cause of death in America, the primary driver of addiction, the root cause of most suicides, and the engine of mass incarceration. With 511,427 annual deaths, 1,401 daily casualties, and millions more suffering among the living, childhood trauma's impact exceeds COVID-19, accidents, and strokes combined.

This is not merely a public health issue—it is a moral crisis. We are allowing nearly six children to be murdered daily while hundreds of thousands of adults die prematurely from preventable childhood wounds. The unseen are not society's shame—they are society's children, and they are calling us to the work we should have done generations ago:

protect children so fiercely that no army of wounded ever marches through our streets again.

The evidence is irrefutable. The deaths are preventable. The only question remaining is whether we have the moral courage to dismantle the machine we have built, to break the cycles we have created, to stop traumatizing children so one day they will no longer fill our morgues, prisons, and streets.

Every 61 seconds, another American dies from childhood trauma.

Two-thirds of these deaths are preventable. Each represents not a moment of weakness but decades of neurobiological destruction that we have the knowledge and tools to prevent. For Michael Kohl, it's too late. For the 50 million American children who will experience trauma before their 18th birthday, it's not.

The evidence is conclusive: Childhood trauma is killing America.

We can prevent it.

We must prevent it.

Anything less is complicity.

The following chapters define in detail the mental, physical, spiritual, and social destruction and disintegration that is the result of a child experiencing trauma. Ultimately, disintegration reflects a profound disturbance in the individual's overall functioning and well-being, affecting their ability to navigate life with stability and resilience.

Chapter Ten

Mental Disintegration

"Trauma results in a fundamental reorganization of the way mind and brain manage perceptions. It changes not only how we think and what we think about, but also our very capacity to think."

–Bessel van der Kolk, M.D.

I'VE READ MANY BOOKS and research papers and have spoken with many mental health professionals on my journey to better understand the impact of childhood trauma. I've attempted without success to understand the difference between a mental illness and a mental disorder. I also struggled to settle on a definition of mental illness. Opinions, dictionaries and reference books differ widely in their definitions. In *Brain Energy*, Dr. Christopher Palmer offers an all-purpose definition of mental illness:

"A mental illness involves changes or abnormalities in emotions, cognition, motivation, and/or behaviors resulting in distress or problems functioning in life."

This makes sense to me. I will adapt this definition for the balance of my book. And correctly or incorrectly, I will use mental illness and mental disorder interchangeably.

The list of disorders, diseases, and dysfunctions linked to adverse childhood experiences (ACEs) is staggering. The sheer magnitude of this disintegration challenges believability, pushing the boundaries of our understanding. I am sure it will also invite skepticism, but we can no longer afford to ignore the compelling evidence that paints a grim portrait of the human condition when trauma invades the formative years.

Trauma is inherently distressing and often unbearable. Survivors of rape, combat veterans, and children who have endured molestation frequently find themselves so overwhelmed by their experiences that they try to suppress these memories, pretending as if nothing occurred in order to forge ahead. Juggling the need for a sense of normalcy while carrying the heavy burdens of fear, shame, and vulnerability requires a tremendous amount of energy.

The desire to heal from trauma is something we all share, but the part of our brain that governs our survival instincts—situated deep within our subconscious—struggles with denial. Even well after a traumatic event has concluded, the slightest suggestion of danger can reignite these survival responses, stimulating off-kilter neural pathways and flooding the body with stress hormones. This reaction often results in uncomfortable emotions, intense physical sensations, or impulsive or aggressive actions. Such responses can be disorienting and overwhelming. As survivors face the turmoil of losing control, they may start to fear that they are irrevocably damaged and beyond hope.

This is not the case.

As we navigate this list—a somber enumeration of the many ways trauma infiltrates and undermines human potential—let us do so with the understanding that these are not mere statistics. They are real lives, with far-reaching implications for individuals, and for society alike. Together, we must confront this reality, for it is only by acknowledging the profound challenges stemming from childhood trauma that we have the opportunity and the responsibility to begin to heal and dismantle the cycles of suffering that persist in our communities.

The burning question is will we look at it or away from it?

What follows is a list of the top 13 major mental illnesses that are linked to early traumatic experiences, along with brief descriptions of their symptoms:

1. Post-Traumatic Stress Disorder (PTSD & Complex PTSD)

The effects of PTSD and complex childhood trauma are very similar and can significantly disrupt a child's emotional, cognitive, and social development. It can hinder their ability to form secure attachments, regulate their emotions, and develop a coherent sense of self. Furthermore, complex trauma can have long-lasting effects into adulthood, contributing to mental health issues, relationship difficulties, and challenges in various aspects of life. The symptoms from PTSD include:

A. **Emotion Dysregulation:** Individuals often struggle to manage their emotions, experiencing intense feelings of anger, sadness, or anxiety that can seem overwhelming or uncontrollable.

B. **Negative Self-Perception:** Those with C-PTSD may have a pervasive sense of worthlessness, guilt, or shame, often stemming from the chronic abuse or neglect they experienced as children.

C. **Difficulty with Relationships:** Establishing and maintaining healthy relationships can be challenging. Individuals may exhibit a fear of abandonment, difficulty trusting others, or patterns of isolation.

D. **Avoidance:** Similar to PTSD, individuals may avoid reminders of the trauma (people, places, conversations) but this can extend to avoiding emotions or experiences that might be associated with their past trauma.

E. **Intrusive Symptoms:** These may include flashbacks or unwanted memories related to the trauma, but are often more varied and less specific than in standard PTSD.

F. **Somatic Symptoms:** Physical manifestations of distress such as chronic pain, fatigue, or other unexplained medical issues can often occur, as the body holds onto trauma.

G. **Dissociation:** A feeling of detachment from oneself or one's surroundings can be common, often serving as a coping mechanism in response to overwhelming stress.

2. Depression

Major depressive disorder can manifest as persistent sadness, loss of interest in activities once enjoyed, changes in appetite or sleep patterns, fatigue, feelings of worthlessness, and difficulty concentrating.

3. Anxiety Disorders

This includes generalized anxiety disorder, panic disorder, and social anxiety disorder. Symptoms can involve excessive worry, restlessness, fatigue, difficulty concentrating, panic attacks, and avoidance of anxiety-provoking situations.

4. Borderline Personality Disorder (BPD)

BPD symptoms include intense emotional instability, impulsive behaviors, distorted self-image, fear of abandonment, and unstable relationships. Individuals may experience intense mood swings and engage in self-harming behaviors.

5. Dissociative Disorders

Symptoms often include detachment from reality, memory loss, a sense of being disconnected from oneself, and experiencing a range of identities or personality states. This can arise as a coping mechanism for trauma.

6. Substance Use Disorders

Individuals may turn to drugs or alcohol as a way to cope with emotional pain stemming from trauma. Symptoms include cravings, inability to control substance use, and continued use despite negative consequences.

7. Reactive Attachment Disorder (RAD)

This disorder is characterized by difficulties in emotional attachments with caregivers. Symptoms may include withdrawal from caregivers, difficulty showing affection or comfort, and problems with self-regulation of emotions.

8. Obsessive-Compulsive Disorder (OCD)

Sufferers may experience intrusive thoughts (obsessions) and feel compelled to perform certain behaviors (compulsions) to alleviate anxiety. Symptoms often disrupt daily functioning and cause significant distress.

9. Eating Disorders

Individuals may develop disorders like anorexia nervosa, bulimia nervosa, or binge eating disorder in an effort to gain control over their circumstances in response to trauma. Symptoms can include extreme weight loss, preoccupation with food, and unhealthy eating behaviors.

10. Attention-Deficit/Hyperactivity Disorder (ADHD)

While ADHD has a biological basis, childhood trauma can exacerbate symptoms such as inattention, hyperactivity, and impulsivity. Trauma may lead to increased difficulties in attention regulation.

11. Hopelessness

Many individuals continue to endure significant suffering long after their initial traumatic experiences. They often find themselves trapped in a cycle of pain and grief, unable to regain a sense of normalcy or move beyond their trauma. This paralysis and hopelessness can stem from the weight of their losses and the persistent emotional anguish they face. Feeling overwhelmed and lacking the necessary support or resources for healing, they struggle to find a way back to a semblance of the life they once knew.

For the majority of people, however, mental disorders don't show themselves in dramatic and easily visible ways. Instead, people suffer alone in silence. They are ashamed. They don't know what to do about their symptoms. Oftentimes, they don't even know they have an illness. They don't think of their symptoms as "symptoms"; they think their suffering is just a natural part of existence. They might believe that they are weak or inferior to others. They may think that they just need to make the most of the life they were given.

Recent research indicates that there is another potential response to hopelessness that current scans are not equipped to detect. Some individuals may enter a state of denial. While their bodies perceive the threat, their conscious minds continue as if nothing is wrong. Even though the mind may become adept at ignoring signals from the emotional brain, the alarm signals persist. The emotional brain remains active, and stress hormones continue to instruct the muscles to either prepare for action or become immobilized. Consequently, the physical repercussions on the organs persist until they manifest as illness, demanding attention. Additionally, medications, drugs, and alcohol can temporarily numb or eliminate these overwhelming sensations and emotions.

S. F. Maier and M. E. Seligman are researchers who introduced the concept of "learned helplessness" through a series of experiments involving dogs.[41] I hesitate to share this research and its learnings, given the cruelty to the animals involved, but I believe the information gained is worth the discomfort. In these studies, the researchers subjected dogs to painful electric shocks while they were confined in locked cages, a scenario they termed "inescapable shock."[42]

After delivering multiple rounds of electric shocks, the researchers opened the doors of the cages and administered shocks again. The control group, which had never experienced shocks, immediately fled the open cages. In stark contrast, the dogs who had previously endured inescapable shock made no attempt to escape, even when the opportunity presented itself. Instead, they lay there whimpering and defecating, resigned to their situation.

This response illustrates a critical point: the simple opportunity to escape does not guarantee that traumatized animals—or people—will choose to seek freedom. Helplessness is a debilitating, sad condition. Like Maier and Seligman's dogs, many individuals who have experienced trauma may simply give up. Rather than explore new possibilities, they remain trapped in familiar fears. Their natural fight-or-flight responses have been suppressed, resulting in either overwhelming agitation or a state of complete collapse.

Sufferers of childhood trauma experience their distress, their symptoms, as an integral part of themselves or their life experiences. Extreme hopelessness may lead the sufferer to no longer want to live.

12. Loss of Imagination

Imagination plays a vital role in enriching our lives. It allows us to transcend the mundane aspects of our daily routines by dreaming about experiences such as travel, delectable food, romance, passion, or having the final say—all the elements that add excitement to our existence. Through imagination, we can create new possibilities; it serves as a critical springboard for bringing our dreams to fruition. It fuels our creative spirit, alleviates feelings of boredom, soothes our pain, heightens our enjoyment, and deepens our most meaningful relationships.

Those sufferers of childhood trauma many times find themselves incessantly drawn back to the past, reminiscing about times of intense engagement and profound emotions. They experience a stagnation of imagination and a reduction in mental adaptability. In the absence of imagination, hope evaporates, the vision of a brighter future diminishes, and the pursuit of aspirations becomes elusive.

13. Suicidality

Childhood trauma is proven to have profound and lasting effects on an individual's mental health and emotional well-being, often leading to an increased risk of suicidal thoughts and behaviors in later life. Experiences such as abuse, neglect, or severe stress during formative years can disrupt emotional development and create feelings of hopelessness and despair. Individuals who have faced childhood trauma may struggle with unresolved feelings of pain, isolation, and low self-worth, making them more vulnerable to mental health challenges.

My brother-in-law Michael is a clear example. Consequently, the psychological scars left by childhood trauma can contribute significantly to a person's risk of considering or attempting suicide, underscoring the need for early intervention and support to address and heal from these traumatic experiences.

While these last three items are more symptoms than mental illnesses, being saddled with a mental illness can result in extreme hopelessness, loss of imagination, and suicidality. This is why I choose to include these under the category of mental disintegration.

Impact of Sexual Abuse

In 1986, researchers Frank Putnam and Penelope Trickett embarked on a groundbreaking study aimed at uncovering the long-term effects of sexual abuse on female development, with a specific focus on girls who endured incest.[43] Notably, prior to this study, insights into the consequences of incest were primarily drawn from retrospective accounts rather than robust evidence. Over a span of 20 years, the research tracked 84 girls with verified histories of sexual abuse and compared their experiences with 82 non-abused peers.

The outcomes of this study revealed alarming trends: girls who had been sexually abused exhibited severe negative effects, including cognitive impairments, depression, dissociation, difficulties in sexual development, increased high school dropout rates, and a higher prevalence of major health issues. Physiologically, these individuals demonstrated anomalies in their stress responses and hormonal profiles, with early onset of puberty and elevated levels of certain hormones.

A particularly compelling element of the study was the contrasting emotional responses observed during assessments. While their non-abused counterparts displayed distress and elevated cortisol levels when faced with stressful inquiries, the abused girls exhibited emotional numbness and significantly reduced cortisol responses over time. This numbing can hinder their ability to identify and address feelings of distress, adversely affecting their social interactions and relationships.

Additionally, the research highlighted a stark difference in the social dynamics of the two groups. Non-abused girls typically formed friendships that fostered emotional and social development, whereas those who experienced sexual abuse grappled with trust issues and low self-esteem, leading to tumultuous relationships with peers. Furthermore, the findings indicated that sexual abuse not only intensified the challenges these girls faced but also expedited their onset of puberty and sexual maturation.

The ramifications of childhood sexual abuse extend beyond immediate trauma, often resulting in unhealthy sexual behaviors because of intertwined psychological, emotional, physiological, and social factors stemming from their traumatic experiences. What follows is a list of critical contributing factors behind this troubling phenomenon.

Sexual Development: Sexual abuse can disrupt normal sexual development, leading to confusion, fear, and anxiety surrounding sex and intimacy. Instead of healthy sexual exploration, the individual may associate sexual activity with trauma, manipulation, and pain.

Self-Perception and Worth: Survivors of sexual abuse frequently struggle with low self-esteem and feelings of worthlessness. To gain a sense of control or validation, they may engage in unhealthy sexual behaviors, including promiscuity, or seek relationships that mimic earlier abusive dynamics.

Numbing and Detachment: Many abused individuals develop coping mechanisms to numb emotional pain, including detachment from their feelings and bodies. Numbing can lead to risky sexual behaviors as the person may not fully engage with the implications of their actions or the emotional consequences of sexual encounters.

Disrupted Trust and Attachment: Experiencing betrayal from a caregiver or trusted adult can severely impact a child's ability to trust others and form healthy attachments. As adults, these survivors might engage in relationships characterized by instability, fear, or hypersexuality, often as a misguided way to seek intimacy or connection.

Reenactment of Trauma: Some survivors might unconsciously reenact their trauma through unhealthy sexual relationships, believing that re-experiencing or controlling the situation can provide closure or understanding of their past. This can lead to a cycle of abusive relationships that perpetuates their trauma.

Lack of Healthy Models and Support: Many survivors lack role models or guidance on establishing healthy relationships and sexual norms. This absence of support can leave them vulnerable to engaging in behaviors that are not conducive to healthy emotional or sexual development.

Psychological Disorders: Sexual abuse is linked to various mental health issues, including depression, anxiety, PTSD, and dissociative disorders. These conditions can distort the survivor's understanding of relationships and sexuality, further contributing to unhealthy patterns.

Cultural and Social Reinforcement: Societal messages about sexuality, particularly regarding women and girls, can play a role in how survivors understand their experiences. Pressure to conform to certain sexual behaviors or stereotypes can shape their sexual patterns in maladaptive ways.

As you can see, the effects of childhood sexual abuse can lead to a complex interaction of emotional, psychological, and social challenges. These challenges can manifest as unhealthy sexual patterns, driven by a need for control, affirmation, or emotional connection, often rooted in the trauma experienced at a young age.

Conduit of Illness: How One Condition Resonates Through the Mind & Body

There are so many dimensions of childhood trauma that make it, in its totality, so grievous and destructive. Each dimension being an unconnected dot. There is so little known about the disorders and disintegration caused by childhood trauma. So many dots yet to be connected and understood.

A survey in the US of more than nine million households reported 68% of people with major depression also met the criteria for an anxiety disorder. Several studies have found that two-thirds of adults with anxiety disorders also met the criteria for major depression.[44] Two researchers took this research much further.

In research examining the relationship between early childhood experiences and adult outcomes, Drs. Avshalom Caspi and Terrie Moffitt found that childhood adversities present risk for most mental disorders including PTSD, depression, anxiety, substance abuse disorders, eating disorders, bipolar disorders, and schizophrenia.[45,46]

If a person has experienced childhood trauma, the most common and earliest disorders that emerge during childhood and adulthood are depression and anxiety. And we now have data that confirms these early disorders serve as pathways to a long list of other mental disorders.

In *Brain Energy*, Dr. Christopher Palmer made the very compelling point that there are many medical disorders that commonly co-occur with mental disorders and vice versa. Some experts have gone so far as to suggest that experiencing childhood trauma creates or opens the common pathway to all mental disorders. We have learned not only do mental disorders have strong bidirectional relationships with one another, many metabolic (physical) and neurological disorders also have strong bidirectional relationships with mental disorders.[20] Many times, those with mental disorders are also associated with higher rates of diabetes. People with schizophrenia are three times more likely to develop diabetes.

What about the flip side? Are those with diabetes more likely to develop mental disorders? The answer is yes. Those with diabetes are two to three times more likely to develop major depression. And, when they get depressed, the depression lasts four times longer than those without diabetes. At any given time, 25% of people with diabetes have clinical depression.

Another study, conducted with data from 1.3 million adolescents, looked at rates of mental disorders over the following 10 years. It was discovered that the adolescents with diabetes were more likely to suffer from a mood disorder, attempt suicide, visit a psychiatrist, or develop any psychiatric disorder.

Based on these findings, it appears it's all connected.

We know that people with mental disorders are more likely to be overweight or obese. One study followed people diagnosed with schizophrenia and bipolar disorder for 20 years. When they were first diagnosed, the majority were not obese. Twenty years later, 62% of those with schizophrenia and 50% of those with bipolar disorder were obese.[47] The obesity rate at the time for all adults in New York State, where the study was conducted, was 27%. Children with autism are 40% more likely to be obese. One meta-analysis of 120 studies found that people with serious mental illness were three times more likely to be obese than people without a mental illness.[48]

Dr. Palmer's work challenges us to make the connections between our psychological experiences and physical health more visible and to foster a comprehensive approach to treatment. By understanding how trauma, mental disorders, and chronic health issues intertwine, we can better understand the even more insidious impact of childhood trauma. Both of which are necessary if we have any hope to drive forward a more integrated and compassionate model of care, ensuring those affected by ACEs receive the holistic support they deserve.

Childhood trauma casts a long shadow on an individual's life, weaving itself into the very fabric of mental health. Research consistently shows that those who endure adverse experiences in their formative years are at a substantially heightened risk for a wide array of mental disorders and illnesses. Conditions such as anxiety, depression, PTSD, and personality disorders are not just possibilities—they are often realities for those grappling with the echoes of their early hardships.

As I have experienced first-hand with my siblings, these echoes of childhood experiences can resonate through our thoughts, perceptions, and emotional responses well into adulthood, illustrating just how profound and destructive trauma can be on the mind. But it doesn't stop there. The repercussions of childhood trauma extend beyond the mental realm, seeping into every aspect of an individual's being. This brings us to the critical discussion of physical disintegration, where we will explore how trauma manifests in the body, influencing health, resilience, and overall well-being.

Join me as we uncover the intricate ways in which our physical selves bear the weight of past experiences. In later chapters we will discuss how the promise of healing can pave the way to restoring both body and mind.

CHAPTER ELEVEN

Physical Disintegration

"The effects of unresolved trauma can be devastating. It can affect our habits and outlook on life, leading to addictions and poor decision-making. It can take a toll on our family life and interpersonal relationships. It can trigger real physical pain, symptoms, and disease. And it can lead to a range of self-destructive behaviors."

–Peter A. Levine, PhD

THE INTERACTION BETWEEN THE mind and body has long been a subject of intrigue, but it was Bessel van der Kolk's groundbreaking work in *The Body Keeps the Score* that illuminated the profound connections between childhood trauma and physical disintegration. In this pivotal book, van der Kolk reveals how traumatic experiences are not merely etched into our memories but are also inscribed in our bodies. He emphasizes that unresolved trauma can lead to a multitude of physical disorders, including chronic pain, autoimmune diseases, and a host of other health complications. We will look closely at the long list of metabolic illnesses that are now known to be linked to childhood trauma. This lens invites us to understand trauma as a holistic experience—one that affects not only our mental well-being but our physical health as well.

The stress and anxiety stemming from early adverse experiences can manifest in tangible ways, altering our physiology, immune function, and overall health. It is crucial to understand that the scars of trauma run deep within the body, influencing our vitality and resilience. By exploring these physical manifestations, we can begin to gain insight into healing pathways that must comprehend and honor both the mind and body, ultimately fostering a more comprehensive approach to recovery. In fact, ACEs and health outcomes are correlated.

We have learned so much from the adverse childhood experiences (ACEs) study. Drs. Anda and Felitti have spawned ongoing studies that have looked at these stressors early in life and their correlation with later health outcomes. A 2017 meta-analysis of 37 such studies looking at 23 health outcomes in more than 250,000 people found that in fact, they are.[15]

The more ACEs a child has, the more likely they are to face poor health outcomes in adulthood. ACEs significantly increase the likelihood of physical inactivity, obesity, and diabetes by 25%-52%. They are also associated with a staggering 266% higher rate of smoking, a 530% increase in the likelihood of developing alcoholism, and a 1,100% increase in the probability of using illegal injectable drugs. Additionally, ACEs contribute to a 450% increase in the chances of engaging in sexual intercourse by age 15 among teenagers.

The influence of ACEs extends to violence as well, leading to over a sevenfold increase in the likelihood of being either a victim or perpetrator of violence, a tenfold increase in problematic drug use, and a thirtyfold increase in suicide attempts. From a physical health perspective, individuals with more than four ACEs face a 220% increased probability of developing liver disease, a 240% higher chance of having chronic obstructive pulmonary disease (COPD), and a 170% increase in the likelihood of experiencing heart disease.

We now know that ACEs clearly affect how long we live. One study of 17,421 people that looked specifically at mortality data estimated that having six or more ACEs takes 20 years off a person's life compared to those with none.[49]

The impact of childhood trauma extends beyond emotional and psychological realms, manifesting in a variety of physical disorders and illnesses that can persist into adulthood. Research has increasingly high-lighted the myriad ways in which unresolved trauma can compromise physical health, leading to conditions that impact daily living and overall quality of life.

When the Lights Go Out: How Trauma Kills the Powerhouses of Life

To understand how childhood trauma creates physical destruction that lasts a lifetime, you need to understand something most people have never heard of: mitochondria. These microscopic structures hold the key to one of the most devastating and previously hidden consequences of childhood trauma—the systematic destruction of our cellular power plants.

Imagine your body as a bustling city, and every building in that city needs electricity to function. Your mitochondria are like thousands of tiny power plants scattered throughout each building, working around the clock to keep the lights on, the elevators running, and all the essential systems operating. When childhood trauma strikes, it's like a coordinated attack on the city's entire electrical grid—one that can leave entire neighborhoods in darkness for decades.

The Invisible Engines of Life

Mitochondria are so small that you could fit about 1,000 of them across the width of a human hair, yet they are quite possibly the most important structures in your body. Most cells contain hundreds or even thousands of these little powerhouses, with your most energy-hungry organs—your brain, heart, and muscles—containing the most.

Think of them as cellular batteries that never stop working. Just like your phone needs a battery to function, every cell in your body needs mitochondria to stay alive and do its job. Their main responsibility is elegantly simple but absolutely crucial: they take the food you eat and the oxygen you breathe and transform them into usable energy called ATP. This process is cellular respiration, and it's literally what keeps you alive.

But mitochondria do far more than just make energy. They're like cellular managers that decide how resources get used throughout your body. Some of your food gets turned into energy, but mitochondria also direct portions to become essential brain chemicals like serotonin, which affects your mood, and dopamine, which influences motivation and pleasure. They control inflammation throughout your body, deciding when to turn your immune response on and off. They respond to stress by sensing what's happening in your environment and adjusting accordingly. They even influence your genes by sending signals that can turn different genetic switches on or off.[50]

The Brain's Electrical Demand

Here's where the story becomes particularly relevant to childhood trauma: your brain is the most energy-demanding organ in your body.

Despite representing only 2% of your body weight, your brain consumes about 20% of your total energy. This means brain cells are absolutely packed with mitochondria—an estimated 200 to 400 billion mitochondria total throughout the human brain.[51]

Individual neurons can contain hundreds to thousands of mitochondria each, with the highest concentrations found at synapses—the connection points between brain cells where thoughts, memories, and emotions are processed. Neurons typically have 10 to 100 times more mitochondria than other cell types because thinking, feeling, and remembering are incredibly energy-intensive processes.[52]

When your mitochondria are healthy and working well, you feel energetic, think clearly, sleep soundly, and generally feel good. Your brain has the power it needs to regulate emotions, process information, form memories, and maintain psychological balance. But when mitochondria become damaged or stop functioning properly, the consequences ripple through every aspect of your mental and physical health.

The Cortisol Catastrophe

This is where childhood trauma enters the picture with devastating consequences. When children experience ongoing stress, fear, abuse, or neglect, their bodies remain in constant "emergency mode." This survival state floods their developing systems with stress hormones, particularly cortisol, which acts like a slow-acting poison to mitochondria.

Under normal circumstances, cortisol serves an important protective function—it mobilizes energy during genuine emergencies. But in traumatized children, the stress response system gets stuck in the "on" position, creating what researchers call "toxic stress." Instead of brief bursts of cortisol during actual threats, these children live with chronically elevated stress hormones that bathe their cells in a corrosive chemical environment.

Cortisol damages mitochondria through multiple pathways. It directly interferes with the cellular machinery that produces ATP, essentially sabotaging the power plants from within. It increases the production of harmful free radicals that attack mitochondrial structures. It disrupts the delicate balance of calcium that mitochondria need to function properly. Most insidiously, chronic cortisol exposure actually causes mitochondria to self-destruct through a process called apoptosis.[53]

Since children's brains and bodies are still developing, this mitochondrial damage occurs during critical windows when neural networks are being established. The result is that traumatized children literally develop with compromised cellular power systems throughout their bodies, but especially in their brains.

When the Power Grid Fails

The consequences of mitochondrial damage from childhood trauma manifest in ways that have puzzled doctors and mental health professionals for decades. Patients present with a constellation of symptoms that seem unrelated but actually reflect the underlying energy crisis in their cells.

Chronic fatigue becomes a defining feature of their lives—not the normal tiredness that comes from exertion, but a bone-deep exhaustion that no amount of rest seems to cure. Their brains, starved of adequate energy, struggle with concentration and memory, creating the cognitive fog that so many trauma survivors describe. Sleep becomes elusive because the cellular systems that regulate circadian rhythms depend on properly functioning mitochondria.

Depression and anxiety often emerge as the brain's energy systems fail to produce adequate neurotransmitters. Without sufficient cellular power, the brain cannot manufacture enough serotonin for mood stability, dopamine for motivation, or GABA for calm. The emotional regulation that requires tremendous neural energy becomes increasingly difficult as mitochondrial function declines.

Perhaps most tragically, **the immune system**—which depends heavily on mitochondrial energy to function—becomes compromised. Traumatized individuals become more susceptible to infections, autoimmune conditions, and inflammatory diseases. Their bodies age faster at the cellular level as damaged mitochondria accelerate the biological aging process.

The Invisible Epidemic

For decades, medical professionals have treated these symptoms as separate conditions requiring different medications and therapies. A patient might see one doctor for chronic fatigue, another for depression, a third for autoimmune problems, and a fourth for sleep disorders—never recognizing that all these symptoms stem from the same root cause: mitochondrial dysfunction initiated by childhood trauma.

This explains why traditional treatments often fall short for trauma survivors. Antidepressants might temporarily boost neurotransmitter levels, but they don't address the underlying energy crisis that prevents the brain from producing adequate neurotransmitters naturally. Stimulants might provide temporary energy, but they further stress already damaged mitochondria. Sleep medications might force unconsciousness, but they don't repair the cellular systems needed for restorative sleep.

The mitochondrial perspective reveals why trauma survivors often say they feel "broken" or that "something is fundamentally wrong" with them. They're not imagining things—there really is something wrong at the most basic cellular level. Their power plants have been damaged, and no amount of willpower, positive thinking, or traditional therapy can repair cellular machinery.

The Intergenerational Transmission

Recent research has revealed an even more disturbing truth: mitochondrial damage from trauma can be passed to the next generation. Unlike nuclear DNA, mitochondria have their own genetic material that is inherited exclusively from mothers. When a woman's mitochondria are damaged by childhood trauma, she can pass that cellular dysfunction to her children.[54]

This helps explain the intergenerational patterns we see in trauma families. Children of traumatized mothers don't just inherit psychological wounds—they inherit compromised cellular energy systems that make them more vulnerable to stress, more prone to mental health problems, and less resilient to life's challenges. The trauma literally becomes embedded in their biology before they're even born.

The Path to Cellular Healing

The story of mitochondrial damage from childhood trauma would be nothing but despair if not for one crucial discovery: mitochondria can be healed and even regenerated throughout life. Unlike many cellular structures, mitochondria have the remarkable ability to repair themselves and multiply when given the right conditions.

This cellular healing happens through a process called mitochondrial biogenesis—the creation of new mitochondria. Regular exercise, particularly strength training and moderate cardiovascular activity, signals the body to produce more mitochondria. Quality nutrition provides the raw materials these cellular powerhouses need to function properly. Restorative sleep gives mitochondria the downtime they require to repair and regenerate.

Perhaps most importantly, addressing trauma through therapy and stress management can reduce the cortisol levels that continue to damage mitochondria throughout life. Practices like meditation, yoga, EMDR, and other trauma therapies don't just heal psychological wounds—they create the internal conditions necessary for cellular recovery.

Certain nutrients specifically support mitochondrial function: CoQ10, which is essential for energy production; magnesium, which mitochondria need for hundreds of enzymatic reactions; B vitamins, which serve as cofactors in energy metabolism; and omega-3 fatty acids, which protect mitochondrial membranes from damage.[55]

Reframing Recovery

Understanding mitochondrial dysfunction reframes the entire conversation about trauma recovery. When trauma survivors struggle with fatigue, brain fog, depression, or physical health problems, they're not being weak or resistant to treatment—they're dealing with real, measurable cellular damage that requires time and specific interventions to heal.

This knowledge also validates the experiences of trauma survivors who have felt dismissed by medical professionals. Their symptoms aren't "all in their head"—they're the result of actual physical changes in how their cells produce energy. The depression, anxiety, and fatigue they experience reflect genuine biological dysfunction at the most fundamental level of cellular life.

Recovery from childhood trauma isn't just about changing thoughts or behaviors—it's about literally rebuilding the cellular infrastructure that trauma destroyed. This process takes time, patience, and a comprehensive approach that addresses both psychological healing and physical restoration.

The mitochondrial lens reveals childhood trauma for what it truly is: not just a psychological wound, but a biological attack on the very foundations of health and vitality. When we understand that trauma kills the powerhouses of life itself, we begin to grasp why its effects are so profound, so persistent, and so devastating across every human function.

Yet this understanding also offers hope. If trauma can damage mitochondria, then healing trauma can restore them. If childhood adversity can dim the lights of cellular life, then safety, nutrition, movement, and therapeutic intervention can turn them back on. The power plants of life are resilient, and with the right conditions, even the deepest cellular wounds can heal.

The human body's capacity for regeneration is remarkable, even after decades of mitochondrial damage. No matter what destruction trauma has caused at the cellular level, supporting mitochondrial health can be a pathway to better physical and mental well-being. It's never too late to start taking care of the powerhouses that take care of you—and in doing so, to reclaim the energy, vitality, and potential that trauma tried to steal.

Key physical disorders and illnesses commonly associated with childhood trauma include:

1. Chronic Pain Syndromes

Chronic pain is a common manifestation of childhood trauma, often taking the form of fibromyalgia, chronic headaches, or back pain. Studies have shown that individuals with a history of trauma may experience heightened sensitivity to pain due to alterations in the body's nervous system and stress response. The mind-body connection plays a significant role here, where unresolved emotional pain can transform into chronic physical pain.

2. Autoimmune Disorders

There is a growing body of evidence linking childhood trauma to autoimmune diseases, such as rheumatoid arthritis, lupus, and multiple sclerosis. As we've learned, trauma can lead to dysregulation of the immune system, resulting in an inflammatory response that mistakenly attacks the body's own tissues. This overactive immune response can set the stage for the development of autoimmune conditions, which are characterized by chronic inflammation and a wide range of symptoms.

3. Cardiovascular Issues

Childhood trauma is associated with an increased risk of cardiovascular diseases, including hypertension, heart disease, and stroke. The stress associated with early trauma can lead to long-term changes in the body's stress response systems, contributing to systemic inflammation and increased blood pressure. Furthermore, behaviors such as smoking, substance abuse, and poor diet—often coping mechanisms for trauma—further exacerbate cardiovascular risk.

4. Gastrointestinal Disorders

Individuals with a history of childhood trauma frequently report gastrointestinal issues, ranging from irritable bowel syndrome (IBS) to more severe conditions like Crohn's disease and ulcers. The gut-brain axis—the bidirectional communication between the gastrointestinal tract and the brain—plays a crucial role here. Stress and trauma can lead to altered gut function, resulting in discomfort, digestive disturbances, and heightened sensitivity to food and stress.

5. Respiratory Problems

Emerging studies suggest a correlation between childhood trauma and respiratory issues, including asthma and chronic obstructive pulmonary disease (COPD). Stress and trauma can lead to increased inflammation in the lungs and heightened bronchial reactivity. Individuals with a trauma history may also be more prone to asthma exacerbations, driven by anxiety and panic attacks.

6. Obesity & Eating Disorders

The relationship between childhood trauma and disordered eating is well-documented. Many individuals use food as a coping mechanism to manage emotional pain, leading to obesity or conditions like anorexia and bulimia. Trauma can disrupt normal eating patterns and trigger changes in metabolism, further complicating weight management and overall health.

7. Sleep Disorders

Dr. Alicia Lieberman, a distinguished child psychologist at the University of California, San Francisco, specializes in child-parent psychotherapy (CPP).[56] Her research has revealed that infants of depressed mothers struggle significantly with sleep regulation; they average about 97 fewer minutes of sleep per night compared to infants of mothers without depression and experience more frequent nighttime awakenings. The impact of childhood adversity on sleep is profound, as it heightens the risk for various sleep disorders, including nightmares, insomnia, narcolepsy, sleepwalking, and even psychiatric-related sleep issues such as sleep-eating.

Quality nighttime sleep is crucial for numerous bodily functions, influencing brain activity, hormonal balance, immune responses, and even DNA transcription. Adequate sleep helps to regulate the hypothalamic-pituitary-adrenal (HPA) axis and the sympathoadrenal medullary (SAM) axis. During sleep, levels of hormones such as cortisol, adrenaline, and noradrenaline decrease, while insufficient sleep is linked to elevated levels of stress hormones, leading to heightened stress reactivity. As discussed in chapter five, these stress hormones initiate a range of biological responses, affecting brain function, hormone levels, the immune system, and genetic activity, ultimately resulting in impairments in cognitive performance, memory, and emotional regulation.

The consequences of sleep deprivation extend beyond feeling tired and irritable; it can also compromise physical health. Lack of adequate sleep has been associated with increased inflammation and a diminished immune response. During sleep, the immune system undergoes essential restorative processes, recalibrating its defenses to effectively combat pathogens. While most people recognize the importance of sleep during illness, it's equally vital for maintaining health during periods of health.

Insufficient sleep diminishes the immune system's ability to fend off the constant exposure to viruses and bacteria.

Furthermore, poor sleep has been linked to decreases in vital hormones, such as growth hormone, and can negatively affect DNA transcription. This is particularly concerning for children, as it may hinder their growth and overall development.

8. Chronic Fatigue Syndrome (CFS)

Chronic Fatigue Syndrome, characterized by profound, unexplained fatigue that doesn't improve with rest, has been linked to a history of trauma. The psychological and physical toll of chronic stress and trauma can overwhelm the body, leading to long-lasting fatigue and an impaired ability to engage in daily activities.

9. Liver Disease (Hepatitis & Jaundice)

Hepatitis refers to inflammation of the liver, which can be caused by viral infections (such as hepatitis A, B, C, D, and E), excessive alcohol consumption, certain medications, and autoimmune diseases. Symptoms may include fatigue, abdominal pain, nausea, vomiting, and, in some cases, jaundice. Chronic hepatitis can lead to long-term liver damage, cirrhosis, and an increased risk of liver cancer.

Jaundice is a condition characterized by the yellowing of the skin and the whites of the eyes, resulting from an accumulation of bilirubin in the bloodstream. Bilirubin is a byproduct of the breakdown of red blood cells and is usually processed by a healthy liver. Jaundice is often a symptom of liver dysfunction, including hepatitis, liver cirrhosis, or bile duct obstruction. It can indicate liver disease and warrants further medical evaluation to determine the underlying cause.

These illnesses don't just happen; they are the result of a disintegration of the body's metabolic systems. Childhood trauma exerts significant influence on both the hormonal and immune systems, creating a cascade of effects that can increase susceptibility to various health risks later in life.

Childhood trauma inflicts lasting damage on the hormonal and immune systems, creating a perfect storm for chronic health risks. Through comprehensive care that targets both the psychological and physiological aftermath of trauma, we can enhance individuals' resilience and ultimately support healthier, more fulfilling living.

Let's take it one step further. What about self-inflicted physical disintegration?

Detrimental habits such as smoking, alcoholism, and illicit drug use are often referred to as "substance use disorders" or "addictive behaviors." More broadly, they can be categorized as "unhealthy coping mechanisms" or "risky behaviors." Many people think these disorders come from a lack of willpower, or from a moral failing. But what if these are frequently employed as First Aid, or methods for coping with stress, trauma, and emotional pain?

An increase in smoking, alcoholism, and illicit drug use in adulthood is closely linked with experiencing childhood trauma and are each associated with a wide range of serious health issues. Below are the possible health implications of these addictive behaviors.

Smoking

Respiratory Diseases: Smoking damages the lungs and airways, leading to chronic obstructive pulmonary disease (COPD), chronic bronchitis, and emphysema.

Cancer: Tobacco use is the leading cause of various cancers, particularly lung cancer, but also cancers of the throat, mouth, esophagus, pancreas, bladder, and kidneys.

Cardiovascular Disease: Smoking increases the risk of heart disease and stroke due to the damage to blood vessels and promotion of atherosclerosis (hardening of the arteries).

Decreased Immune Function: The toxins in cigarettes can suppress immune system functions, leading to increased susceptibility to infections.

Reproductive Issues: Smoking can lead to fertility problems in both men and women and is associated with complications during pregnancy, such as low birth weight and preterm birth.

Alcoholism

Liver Disease: Chronic alcohol consumption can lead to liver problems such as fatty liver, alcoholic hepatitis, fibrosis, and cirrhosis.

Mental Health Disorders: Alcoholism is often linked to mental health issues such as depression, anxiety, and increased risk of suicide. It can also exacerbate existing mental illnesses.

Cardiovascular Problems: Excessive alcohol intake can lead to high blood pressure, cardiomyopathy (disease of the heart muscle), and increased risk of heart attack and stroke.

Cancer Risk: Alcohol consumption is linked to an elevated risk of several cancers, including breast, liver, colorectal, and esophageal cancer.

Neurological Damage: Long-term alcoholism can lead to cognitive impairments, memory issues, and neurological disorders such as Wernicke-Korsakoff syndrome (severe memory disorders).

Illicit Drug Use

Addiction and Dependency: Many illicit drugs can lead to physical and psychological dependence, causing severe withdrawal symptoms and cravings.

Mental Health Issues: Drug abuse is closely linked to mental health disorders, including anxiety, depression, and psychosis. Some substances can exacerbate existing mental health conditions or lead to new ones.

Infectious Diseases: Intravenous drug use can increase the risk of infectious diseases such as HIV/AIDS and hepatitis C due to needle sharing.

Cardiovascular Issues: Certain drugs can cause severe cardiovascular problems, including heart attacks and arrhythmias. Stimulants, such as cocaine and methamphetamine, are particularly harmful to the heart.

Respiratory Problems: Smoking illicit drugs, such as marijuana or crack cocaine, can lead to respiratory diseases similar to those caused by tobacco.

It is widely recognized that drug and alcohol use can lead to mental health disorders, and conversely, individuals with mental health conditions are more likely to engage in substance use. Consider the young man who smokes excessive amounts of marijuana and develops schizophrenia, the alcoholic who experiences dementia, or the cocaine user with bipolar disorder. Many tend to believe these outcomes result solely from the harmful effects of drugs on the brain, or that these individuals had underlying predispositions toward mental illness that drugs exacerbated. Both interpretations hold some truth, but the exact mechanisms behind this relationship have remained unclear—until now.

Brain Energy presents findings that shed light on this connection, suggesting that drugs and alcohol impact metabolic processes. Some individuals turn to drugs and alcohol because they are already facing metabolic challenges, such as depression, anxiety, or other distressing feelings. In their search for relief, they may resort to substances. Generally, those experiencing symptoms related to underactive brain cells—common in depression—might seek stimulants to feel more energized.

Conversely, individuals with symptoms linked to overactive brain cells, such as anxiety or psychosis, might use sedatives to calm their heightened states. If a particular substance provides relief, it's easy to see how one could become dependent on it. In their pursuit of feeling "better," some might not actually feel improved; they may just feel "different"—perhaps numb or detached from reality. For some, this altered state can be preferable to their usual emotional state. This cycle of seeking substance use as a coping mechanism likely contributes to the higher prevalence of substance use disorders among those with mental health conditions.

Each of these habits poses significant health risks that can lead to chronic disease, diminished quality of life, and even premature death. If a person who was exposed to childhood trauma who also smoked for 30 years dies of lung cancer, did that person die from the tobacco or the trauma? No matter your answer, childhood trauma has the potential to initiate a convoluted downward spiral.

Stating the obvious, it is important for individuals struggling with these behaviors to seek help through medical and psychological support to mitigate these health risks and have a shot at recovery.

In summary, the possible physical disintegration stemming from childhood trauma encompasses a wide array of disorders and illnesses. While it is a shocking statistic, we can all begin to understand why those who have experienced more than six ACEs die 20 years too early. As research continues to reveal these connections, it becomes increasingly clear that effective healing must address not just the mind but also the body. Understanding the physical repercussions of childhood trauma can guide therapeutic interventions, paving the way for integrative approaches that promote holistic recovery and well-being.

Of all the devastating physical consequences of childhood trauma we've explored in this chapter, none is more final than premature death. This isn't just about reduced quality of life or managing chronic conditions—it's about lost decades, stolen futures, and empty chairs at family gatherings.

The research is heartbreaking but clear: if you experience six or more Adverse Childhood Experiences, you're likely to die nearly 20 years earlier than someone who grew up in safety.[49] Twenty years. That's not just a statistic—that's grandchildren never known, retirement dreams never realized, wisdom never shared. It's life, cut brutally short.

I've witnessed this ultimate cost firsthand. My brothers Adam and Patrick never made it to old age—their struggles with addiction, born from childhood wounds, took them decades before their time. They weren't just statistics in a research paper; they were beloved sons, brothers, and friends whose futures were stolen by the biological cascade that began in childhood.

The path from childhood trauma to early death isn't mysterious—it's mapped out in our cells and systems. Your body literally turns against itself as autoimmune diseases like lupus, MS, and rheumatoid arthritis attack your organs from within.[57] The constant inflammation from childhood stress damages your blood vessels, restricts circulation, and slowly suffocates your tissues.[58,59,60] As Dr. Bessel van der Kolk reminds us, these reactions "are not the result of moral failings or signs of lack of willpower or bad character—they are caused by actual changes in the brain."

The Dunedin researchers showed us that this inflammation can be measured, tracked over decades as it damages organs and systems throughout the body.[19] Dr. Christopher Palmer's work in *Brain Energy* explains how these changes reduce brain cell function, affecting everything from sleep to motivation.[20]

And when the pain becomes too much to bear, many turn to self-medication—alcohol, cigarettes, drugs—creating a second wave of physical destruction. The numbers are staggering: those with four or more ACEs are over 11 times more likely to inject drugs, nine times more likely to attempt suicide, and five times more likely to develop alcoholism compared to those without trauma histories.

Even our natural defenses fail us. The immune system, worn down by years of stress hormones and dysregulated cortisol (as shown in Bruce and Fisher's landmark research), can no longer clear away the cancer cells our bodies naturally produce.[61] Tumors grow where they once would have been destroyed.

This isn't just body breakdown—it's whole-person disintegration. This book explores the mental, spiritual, and social fragmentation, but this physical destruction is the most final. You can't heal a body that's no longer here.

I think about Adam and Patrick every day.

What would they be doing now?

What conversations would we be having?

What joys would they be experiencing?

These aren't just philosophical questions—they represent the concrete reality of lives cut short by trauma's biological cascade.

The most tragic part? These deaths are preventable. The biological pathways from childhood trauma to early death are becoming clearer through research by scientists like Tottenham and colleagues, who showed physical changes in the amygdalae of children who experienced severe neglect. Dr. Alicia Lieberman's work on child-parent psychotherapy offers hope for healing these wounds early, before the physical deterioration begins.

As we close this chapter on physical disintegration, remember that the 20-year gap isn't inevitable.[49] It's a call to action—to prevent childhood trauma where possible, to intervene early when it occurs, and to support healing at any stage. Because no one should lose decades of life to wounds inflicted in childhood.

And to Adam and Patrick: Your stories matter. They're helping others understand what happens when childhood trauma goes unhealed. I couldn't save you, but I pray and hope your experiences will help save others from similar fates.

Chapter Twelve

Spiritual Disintegration

"Healing from childhood trauma is not merely about restoration; it is a journey toward reclaiming the soul that was lost in the shadows of suffering."

–Unknown

It's well documented that spirituality can play a significant role in healing from trauma, often enhancing the likelihood of recovery. Many individuals find that connecting with a deeper sense of purpose, faith, or community provides a framework for understanding and processing their experiences. Spiritual practices—such as meditation, prayer, or mindfulness—can cultivate a sense of inner peace, fostering resilience in the face of adversity. Ironically, we now know that experiencing childhood trauma also has the effect of turning the sufferer away from God and spirituality.

Childhood trauma can leave profound scars on the psyche, influencing an individual's worldview and belief systems. For many who suffer from traumatic experiences in their formative years, spirituality and faith often become significantly affected. A common sentiment shared by those grappling with the aftermath of such trauma is the struggle to reconcile their suffering with the existence of a benevolent God. In fact, the question often arises: "How can there be a God? If there were, He would never have allowed this trauma to happen to me." This poignant inquiry encapsulates a broader struggle faced by many trauma survivors, as they grapple with feelings of abandonment, betrayal, and existential doubt.

For children, experiences of abuse, neglect, or emotional trauma can disrupt their understanding of safety and love. These formative experiences shape their perception of the world as a place that is unpredictable and fraught with danger. In a typically nurturing environment, the idea of a protective, loving deity serves to provide comfort and solace to young minds. However, when trauma occurs, it can shatter that foundational belief. Children may internalize the notion that if a higher power existed, it would intervene in moments of suffering. The absence of divine intervention can lead to feelings of abandonment, reinforcing the belief that God is indifferent to their pain or, worse, complicit in their suffering.

The crisis of faith that often follows childhood trauma can manifest in a complete rejection of spiritual beliefs. The emotional turmoil and confusion resulting from traumatic events can cause individuals to distance themselves from any sense of spirituality. Where once there may have been a sense of hope and trust in a higher power, there is now a pervasive sense of betrayal. As survivors process their trauma, they may adopt a worldview that categorically denies or questions the existence of a compassionate God. This disillusionment can be particularly acute for those who were raised in religious contexts that emphasized the importance of faith and divine protection.

The individual journey away from spirituality can be incredibly lonely and fraught with internal conflict. Survivors may experience feelings of guilt for abandoning their faith, yet the weight of their trauma breeds resentment towards the very idea of a loving deity. This tension can become a source of significant psychological distress. They may find themselves longing for a connection to something greater, but their trauma prevents them from feeling safe in such an embrace. The cognitive dissonance is profound: How can one reconcile the notion of a loving God with the reality of their suffering?

Despite the profound impact of childhood trauma on spiritual beliefs, it is essential to recognize that healing and reconnection with spirituality can occur, albeit often through a nuanced and complex journey. Some individuals find solace in exploring spirituality on their terms, seeking a connection to the divine that aligns more closely with their personal experiences rather than traditional religious frameworks. This journey may involve redefining one's understanding of God—not as an omnipotent being who protects from suffering, but as a source of comfort and strength who walks alongside them in their pain.

Therapeutic practices can also play a crucial role in this process. Spirituality, intertwined with healing modalities, encourages individuals to confront their trauma and explore the depths of their beliefs. Through therapy, they can begin to rebuild a sense of safety and trust, which may eventually extend to their understanding of spirituality and faith.

Humans have an intrinsic drive to seek purpose, which seems to be embedded in our neurological makeup. This fundamental need for meaning is closely linked to both metabolic and mental health. When you combined what we have discussed here related to depression, hopelessness and lack of spirituality, you can easily arrive to the conclusion that those who have experienced childhood trauma could easily develop a lack of purpose. When individuals lack a sense of purpose, it makes everything worse by creating even more of a chronic stress response, which can lead to a range of negative mental and health consequences.

Research on the significance of life's purpose is ongoing, revealing strong correlations with various health outcomes. It's not surprising that a diminished sense of purpose is linked to depression, as the feelings of hopelessness often compound one another in a cyclical, downward pattern. However, the repercussions of a lack of purpose extend beyond mental health; they also encompass metabolic disorders and affect longevity.

For instance, a study involving nearly 7,000 adults aged 51 to 61 in the US found that those with the lowest sense of purpose were approximately 2.5 times more likely to experience premature mortality compared to their counterparts who reported a strong sense of purpo se.[62] They also produced more evidence that those experiencing six or more ACEs before age 18 will die 20 years to soon. This highlights the critical role that having a meaningful direction for our life plays in our overall health and well-being.

Bleeding in the Pews

The Greatest Public Health Crisis in American History is Hiding in Our Churches—And We Can Help Stop It

Every Sunday, sanctuaries fill with voices lifted in praise, hands raised toward heaven. The hymns ring out with hope, the prayers ascend with faith, and the sermons proclaim God's love and healing power. But beneath this beautiful hum of worship, a devastating truth pulses through our pews: The majority of the people singing, praying, and seeking God carry invisible wounds so deep they've become the leading cause of death in our nation.

Seven out of 10 adults in American churches are trauma sufferers and survivors. They sit among us, bearing neurobiological scars from childhood experiences so damaging they continue to kill 1,401 Americans every single day. These wounds cost our country $14 trillion annually and have become the number one cause of addiction, suicide, and incarceration in America.

Yet most of our shepherds don't understand the depths of their flock's bleeding.

This isn't just another ministry challenge. This is America's greatest crisis hiding in plain sight—and our churches hold the key to healing a nation. But first, we must stop pretending that prayer alone will heal neurobiological damage and start understanding that we're in the fight of our lives for the souls of our people.

The crisis in our churches is so profound that I have written an entire book dedicated to this subject. In *Bleeding in the Pews: The Church's Kairos Moment*, I explore in depth how churches can become trauma-responsive sanctuaries capable of true healing.

The War Against the Human Heart

Behind the Sunday service smiles sit trauma survivors whose childhoods were marked by experiences that literally rewired their nervous systems. The grandmother who flinches when voices are raised during passionate worship. The deacon whose hands shake during communion because touch still feels dangerous. The Sunday school teacher who can't explain why she feels unsafe in her own sanctuary despite decades of faithful service.

These responses aren't spiritual weaknesses—they're neurobiological adaptations to overwhelming childhood stress. When we tell these wounded souls to "pray harder" or "have more faith," we're not just missing the mark. We're deepening wounds that are already destroying lives.

Jamie's Story: When Faith Isn't Enough

Let me tell you about my brother Jamie—a man whose story reveals why our churches must learn to see what they've been missing.

Jamie is a man of deep, authentic faith. His relationship with God is real, personal, and unwavering. He knows Scripture, has served faithfully in multiple ministries, and trusts completely in God's power. Yet for decades, Jamie lived with a persistent undercurrent of depression and anxiety that never quite went away.

It wasn't debilitating. Jamie functioned well—built a successful career, raised a family, led Bible studies, prayed beautiful prayers that moved others to tears. From the outside, no one would have known anything was wrong. But Jamie knew. Something was off. A low-grade heaviness that colored everything. An anxiousness that never fully lifted. He could manage it, push through it, live with it—but it was always there, like background noise he'd learned to ignore but could never quite silence.

He did what faithful people do. He prayed. He claimed promises. He memorized verses about peace and joy. He never stopped believing God could heal him. The church offered him everything it knew how to give.

The medical route proved equally frustrating. Doctor after doctor prescribed medication after medication, but nothing seemed to address what was actually wrong. Jamie kept searching, kept praying, kept hoping.

Then his younger brother—that's me—started researching childhood trauma for a memoir about our shared upbringing. As I shared what I was learning, Jamie began to wonder: Could his lifelong struggle be connected to what happened in our childhood? Not a spiritual failure, but a neurobiological wound?

He found a Christian therapist who specialized in trauma recovery and began EMDR therapy—Eye Movement Desensitization and Reprocessing.

After just seven sessions, Jamie experienced dramatic improvement. Not a magical cure—healing is rarely that simple—but a breakthrough that thirty years of prayer and medication hadn't produced. The persistent heaviness began to lift. The anxiety that had shadowed him for decades lost its grip. For the first time, Jamie felt like he was actually healing, not just coping.

Today, Jamie continues on his journey of healing and thriving. He's become an outspoken advocate for therapy within the church, wanting others to know what he didn't know for three decades: Childhood trauma creates real wounds in the brain, and those wounds often need specialized care to heal—care that complements faith, not replaces it.

Jamie's story reveals a gap in our ministry: We're equipped to address spiritual struggles but often blind to neurobiological ones. How many years might have been different if just one person in our church had understood how childhood trauma affects the brain?

How many more Jamies are sitting in our sanctuaries right now, faithfully praying, quietly struggling, waiting for someone to help them see what's actually wrong?

The Four Wounds That Destroy Lives

When childhood trauma strikes, it doesn't just hurt—it systematically disintegrates people across four devastating dimensions that traditional ministry completely misses:

Mental Disintegration

Depression, anxiety, PTSD, and other mental health conditions aren't spiritual problems—they're neurobiological injuries that need informed care alongside prayer. When childhood trauma rewires the developing brain, it creates patterns of hypervigilance and emotional chaos that make receiving God's peace nearly impossible through traditional means alone. The stress hormones of cortisol and adrenaline continue to flow even when no danger is present. This excess of stress hormones kills precious mitochondria in the brain and begins the creation of mental disorders and illness. Mental disorders create pathways to metabolic diseases.

Physical Disintegration

The body literally keeps the score of childhood trauma. Chronic pain, autoimmune disorders, heart disease, diabetes—conditions that fill our prayer request lists—often trace back to adverse childhood experiences. The stress hormones of trauma destroy mitochondria in both brain and body, creating the very illnesses that plague our congregations.

Societal Disintegration

Trauma destroys the ability to trust and connect—the very foundation of Christian fellowship. Survivors often appear "difficult" or "resistant" when they're actually protecting nervous systems stuck in survival mode. This isolation prevents them from experiencing the healing community that could demonstrate God's love.

Spiritual Disintegration

This cuts deepest of all. When trauma survivors ask, "How can there be a God? If there were, He would never have allowed this to happen to me," they're not having a crisis of faith—they're having a crisis of safety. Their wounded spirits cannot receive love from a God they cannot trust, not because of spiritual failure, but because of neurobiological damage.

The Heartbreaking Question: "How Can There Be a God?"

Every minister will face this moment: a trauma survivor sits across from you, tears streaming, asking the question that reveals the depth of evil's impact: "How can there be a God when this happened to me?"

Maybe it's the woman whose father abused her for years while she prayed every night for it to stop. Perhaps it's the sibling who watched his three-month-old brother die after being thrown against a wall—four days of agony before death finally came. Or the countless adults discovering that their childhood pain wasn't just bad memories but wounds that continue killing Americans daily.

This question isn't theological curiosity—it's the cry of a soul whose capacity to trust has been shattered at the neurobiological level. When we offer simplistic answers like "God has a plan" or "Everything happens for a reason," we're not providing comfort. We're adding salt to wounds that run deeper than words can reach.

The truth is more complex and more beautiful than easy answers allow.

Understanding the Mystery of Suffering

When children experience trauma, their developing brains adapt to survive overwhelming evil. These adaptations affect every aspect of their being—mental, physical, social, and spiritual. The enemy of souls targets childhood precisely because these are the years when our capacity to trust and receive love is formed.

But here's what sustains faith through the darkest questions: God doesn't stand apart from human anguish—He enters it fully. When Christ wept over Lazarus, when He cried out "My God, my God, why have You forsaken me?" on the cross, we see that our God absorbs into Himself every moment of agony that every abused child has ever experienced.

That three-month-old baby who died after being thrown against a wall was not alone in his suffering. The same Jesus who wept over Jerusalem was present with that child, feeling every moment of terror and pain. The mystery that keeps faith alive isn't why God allows evil, but how a God who experiences every moment of that baby's agony with perfect intensity doesn't immediately destroy every perpetrator of such acts.

The Sacred Nature of Doubt

When trauma survivors express doubt about God's goodness, they're not exhibiting spiritual failure—they're demonstrating their souls' refusal to accept evil without a fight. Their questions reveal hearts that take both suffering and divine love seriously enough to wrestle with the profound mysteries of existence.

This kind of doubt actually honors God more than simple belief that has never been tested. It represents the wrestling of Jacob, the laments of David, the questions of Job—honest cries that ultimately deepen rather than destroy faith.

Every moment of uncertainty a trauma survivor feels when confronted with evil is preparing them to become ministers to others whose faith has been shattered. Their willingness to doubt, to struggle, to refuse easy answers makes them trustworthy to those whose trust has been utterly betrayed.

When someone who has wrestled with these impossible questions finally sits across from another trauma survivor, they won't offer platitudes. They'll offer the wrestling of their own soul, the hard-won faith that emerges not from easy answers but from refusing to let go of God even in the darkness.

The doubt isn't their enemy—it's their teacher.

The Shepherds Who Cannot See the Wounds

Here's our most devastating failure: most seminary programs contain little to no training on trauma-informed ministry. Our pastors, no matter how well-intentioned or spiritually mature, are attempting to heal trauma survivors without understanding the neurobiological realities of their condition.

It's like sending doctors to treat cancer without teaching them oncology, then wondering why their patients remain sick despite receiving encouragement and prayer.

But the problem runs deeper than inadequate training. Before we can heal our congregations, our ministry leaders need to tend to their own wounds instead of focusing on others while their own hearts' wounds are still hemorrhaging over those they are trying to help.

Statistics suggest that 70% of our ministry leaders carry their own unhealed trauma. When emotionally wounded leaders encounter traumatized congregants, the result is often re-traumatization rather than healing. Leaders with unresolved wounds, often elevated precisely because they're compelling speakers who can draw crowds, can create systems that are systematically destructive while hiding behind Christian language.

This is why church hurt is epidemic. Wounded leaders create wounded systems that wound people who are already wounded. The cycle continues until someone has the courage to say: "This must stop."

The Transformation Churches Must Embrace

The solution isn't to abandon faith—it's to enhance our ministry with trauma-informed understanding that recognizes how God designed the human brain and nervous system to heal. Every church must become trauma-informed, and this transformation requires:

Leadership Healing First

Ministry teams must address their own trauma before attempting to heal others. This isn't optional—it's essential for preventing further harm. It is certainly more difficult for wounded healers to provide safe healing environments.

Trauma Awareness Training

All leaders need basic understanding of how adverse childhood experiences affect brain development, emotional regulation, and spiritual receptivity. We don't need to become therapists, but we must recognize trauma symptoms and understand why traditional approaches at times fall short.

Safety-First Environments

Worship and ministry must signal safety to hypervigilant nervous systems rather than triggering fight-or-flight responses. This means understanding how volume, lighting, physical proximity, and even theological language can re-traumatize wounded people.

Professional Partnerships

Churches need relationships with trauma-informed Christian therapists who understand both neurobiological and spiritual dimensions of healing. When someone like Jamie needs specialized care, we must be ready to connect them with qualified help. The church needs the science of public health and public health needs the true source of hope and healing found in the church.

Long-Term Commitment to Healing

Healing trauma requires consistent, patient presence over time, not quick fixes or breakthrough moments. Real transformation happens through small, consistent acts of love and safety that slowly rebuild trust.

The Biblical Mandate We Cannot Ignore

Scripture commands us to "be wise as serpents and gentle as doves." Wisdom demands that we understand the wounds we're called to heal. When Jesus encountered the demon-possessed man among the tombs,

He didn't offer a quick prayer—He engaged with the complex trauma presentation before Him, understanding that healing required more than spiritual intervention alone.

The same God who designed our brains to adapt to trauma also designed them to heal through safe, loving relationships. Recent neuroscience research confirms what people of faith have always believed: transformation is possible. The brain's neuroplasticity means the same organ that adapted to trauma can adapt to safety and love.

But this healing requires what trauma researcher Robert Stolorow calls "finding a relational home where intense emotional pain can be held." Churches should be the ultimate relational home for traumatized souls. Today they are not.

The Promise That Sustains Hope

Here's the message of hope for every trauma survivor wrestling with impossible questions: trauma responses are not permanent. The brain that was wounded can be healed. The heart that learned to fear love can learn to receive it. The spirit that was crushed can be restored.

But this healing requires what I call "the presence of mature love"—sustained, informed, compassionate relationships that provide both neurobiological and spiritual safety necessary for souls to risk trusting again.

When churches learn to provide this kind of informed love, miracles happen. Not just spiritual transformation, but neurobiological healing that allows people to finally experience the God they've always longed to know.

The Greatest Ministry Opportunity of Our Time

The epidemic of childhood trauma represents both our greatest pastoral challenge and our most profound ministry opportunity. When we learn to recognize and respond to trauma with both spiritual wisdom and scientific understanding, our churches can become what they were always meant to be: true sanctuaries of healing.

As Isaiah promised: "He has sent me to bind up the brokenhearted, to proclaim freedom for the captives and release from darkness for the prisoners" (Isaiah 61:1).

Churches should be the first aid stations for trauma, not the places that perpetuate it.

Every Sunday, approximately 70% of our congregations sit bleeding in the pews while we offer solutions that cannot reach their wounds. Sometimes miracles heal instantly—and we celebrate those testimonies. But millions more suffer like Jamie did for 30 years because no one in the church understood that their anxiety, depression, and spiritual struggles were trauma symptoms, not spiritual failures.

These wounded souls deserve better than our ignorance. They deserve churches that understand both the science and the sacred, that can minister to neurobiological wounds and spiritual hunger with equal wisdom.

A Call to Revolutionary Love

The bleeding in our pews is real. The solution is within our reach. The time to act is now.

It's time to stop asking traumatized people to have more faith and start asking ourselves why we've failed to create the safe, healing communities they desperately need. We need systems of support and cultures of care. We need community care even more than self-care. It's time to stop treating trauma symptoms as spiritual problems and start understanding the neurobiological realities of the wounds we're called to heal.

It's time to transform our churches from places that unknowingly wound the wounded into sanctuaries that counter evil's assault with informed, revolutionary love.

This transformation begins with a simple recognition: The person sitting next to you in church may be fighting the battle of their life against wounds they didn't choose and can't simply pray away. They need more than our prayers—they need our understanding. They need more than our faith—they need our wisdom. They need more than our good intentions—they need our informed love.

The enemy may wound in childhood, but our God specializes in healing the brokenhearted. When we learn to be His instruments of both spiritual and neurobiological restoration, we become part of the most important healing ministry in human history.

The choice is ours. Will we continue ministering in ignorance while our people suffer in silence? Or will we finally become the trauma-informed sanctuaries that can stop the bleeding and begin the healing our wounded world desperately needs?

The bleeding in our pews is real. The healing can be, too.

The journey from trauma to healing is deeply personal and complex. Childhood experiences of trauma often create a chasm between the sufferer and their spirituality, casting shadows of doubt on the existence of a benevolent God.

The struggle with faith is not merely a question of belief but a profound dialogue with one's own pain and the search for meaning in a world that often feels chaotic and cruel. While many may initially turn away from spirituality in the aftermath of trauma, the path toward healing can also lead to a renewed understanding of spirituality—one that acknowledges suffering yet embraces hope, connection, and the possibility of transformation.

Churches that have an understanding of the neurological complexities and needs of those who have experienced childhood trauma have the real potential to deliver the transformation and peace so vital to the sufferer's healing.

Chapter Thirteen

Social Disintegration

"In the silent echoes of childhood trauma, the bonds of connection fray, leaving a tapestry of society torn by isolation, mistrust, and unspoken pain."

–Michael Menard

THE PREVIOUS CHAPTERS ON mental, physical, and spiritual disintegration have primarily highlighted the struggles of the individual. Those disintegrations serve as precursors to a broader social disintegration that affects all of humanity. When multiple individuals within a community experience these forms of disintegration, the fabric of societal cohesion begins to unravel. Communities may become fragmented, empathy and understanding can erode, and systemic issues such as poverty, violence, and inequality become more pronounced.

Furthermore, as families and support networks are tested by the fallout of trauma, the collective ability to foster healthy relationships and community resilience diminishes. Disintegration at the individual level thus sets in motion a cycle that can manifest in societal dysfunction—exacerbating issues such as mental health crises, substance abuse, crime, and community alienation.

When individuals who have experienced childhood trauma are trapped in survival mode, their focus shifts to defending against perceived threats, leaving little room for nurturing, care, and love. For these individuals, this state of constant vigilance competes with their ability to form and maintain close relationships, as well as their capacity to imagine, plan, engage in play, learn, and attend to the needs of others.

Feeling safe with those around us is perhaps the most critical component of mental health. Secure connections form the foundation for meaningful and fulfilling lives. Unfortunately, many survivors of trauma find themselves frequently out of sync with their peers and loved ones.

Ultimately, those who have faced childhood trauma—including neglect, abuse, and family dysfunction—experience both subtle and significant separations from society. This disconnection robs them of one of the most vital elements of a healthy and happy existence: meaningful, trusting relationships. This isolation is in my opinion the most significant aspect of social disintegration experienced by those who have been exposed to childhood trauma. Following is a partial list of the dimensions that in their totality contribute to this force that is greater than gravity and is pulling down humanity.

1. 70% of All Adults in the US Suffer from Childhood Trauma

A staggering proportion of adults in the US carry the burden of childhood trauma, which can manifest as mental health issues, relationship difficulties, and coping mechanisms that often lead to destructive behaviors. This widespread trauma creates a cycle of distress that not only affects individuals but also spills over into families and communities. As trauma survivors struggle to form healthy relationships, social cohesion erodes, contributing to increased isolation and a lack of mutual support in society.

2. Impact of Tobacco, Alcohol, & Illegal Drugs

"I have absolutely no pleasure in the stimulants in which I sometimes so madly indulge. It has not been in the pursuit of pleasure that I have periled life and reputation and reason. It has been in the desperate attempt to escape from torturing memories."

–Edgar Allan Poe

Substance abuse is often used as a coping mechanism to alleviate the pain associated with trauma. However, tobacco, alcohol, and illegal drugs can further exacerbate mental and physical health issues, leading to a range of social problems. The consequences of addiction can ripple through families, destabilizing homes and increasing healthcare costs. Moreover, substance abuse often correlates with higher incidences of violence, accidents, and crime, fundamentally undermining community safety and well-being.

According to the National Institute on Drug Abuse (NIDA) and the Substance Abuse and Mental Health Services Administration (SAMH-SA), millions of Americans use illegal drugs each year. In 2021, approximately 50 million Americans (around 18% of the population) reported using illicit drugs, which includes marijuana, cocaine, heroin, methamphetamine, and other substances. Let's drill down into the specifics that create social disintegration:

A. Health Consequences

The use of illegal drugs often leads to severe health issues, including addiction, mental illness, and chronic diseases. Substance abuse can result in a range of physical health problems, such as heart disease, respiratory issues, and infectious diseases that can arise from needle sharing. Mental health complications, including depression, anxiety, and psychosis, can also stem from drug use, creating a cycle of despair that not only affects the individual but also places a burden on healthcare systems.

B. Family Disruption

Illegal drug use can lead to significant instability within families. Parents who struggle with addiction may have difficulty providing the care and support that their children need, leading to neglect and emotional trauma. This disruption can create an environment that fosters further substance abuse among the next generation, perpetuating cycles of dysfunction and instability.

C. Crime & Safety Issues

The illegal drug trade is intertwined with crime. Drug trafficking, gang violence, and theft often escalate as individuals and organizations vie for control of lucrative markets. Communities plagued by drug-related crime experience decreased safety, which can lead to heightened fear and isolation among residents. The resulting environment of lawlessness can deter investment and development, further marginalizing already vulnerable neighborhoods.

D. Economic Costs

The economic impact of illegal drugs and alcoholism is staggering. It's estimated that the cost to treat the disorders and disease brought on by childhood trauma is $14.1 trillion per year, which includes losses from decreased productivity. The costs associated with healthcare, law enforcement, and social services required to address addiction, and its consequences can strain public resources. Lost productivity due to addiction, absenteeism, and premature death also contributes to decreased economic output, impacting families and communities. The financial burden can divert funds from essential services, such as education and infrastructure, exacerbating social inequalities.

E. Social Fragmentation

Illegal drug use can erode social trust and cohesion within communities. Neighborhoods grappling with drug problems often see an increase in stigma, leading to social isolation of affected families and individuals. This breakdown in community bonds diminishes the collective capacity to support one another, making it harder to combat other social issues and undermining civic engagement.

F. Impact on Youth

The presence of illegal drugs in communities poses significant risks to young people, who may be more susceptible to experimentation and addiction. Early exposure to drugs can lead to a host of negative outcomes, including poor academic performance, behavioral issues, and an increased likelihood of involvement in the criminal justice system. The long-term effects can hinder the potential of an entire generation.

G. Harm to Self & Others

Dr. Gabor Maté, a physician who works with drug addicts, reports that early traumatic experiences are stored in people's brains and bodies and are daily "acted out" in the form of violence toward others or "acted in," in the form of self-harming beliefs and behaviors.[63] This manifestation of trauma isn't random; it's the brain's desperate attempt to cope with overwhelming pain. When childhood trauma remains unresolved, the survivor often turns to substances or violence as a form of self-medication—either to numb the pain or to externalize it.

Aggression toward others often represents an unconscious reenactment of their own trauma, while self-destructive behaviors can stem from deep-seated feelings of worthlessness and shame implanted during their traumatic experiences. As Dr. Maté explains, what we label as addiction is not simply a matter of choice or moral failing, but rather an attempt to escape the unbearable sensations and emotions stored in the traumatized body.

3. Fatherless Homes

Childhood trauma contributes to a larger, generational issue, including shaping family dynamics and can contribute to the occurrence of fatherless homes. The effects of trauma on mental health, relationships, and socioeconomic stability can cascade through generations, influencing the likelihood of future family disruptions. One of the more significant ramifications is its contribution to the prevalence of fatherless homes. This occurs through several interrelated mechanisms.

Firstly, trauma often leads to a breakdown in family dynamics. Parents who experience childhood trauma may struggle with mental health issues, such as depression or substance abuse, which can impair their ability to maintain healthy relationships, including with their partners. This dysfunction can result in increased conflict, separation, or divorce, ultimately leading to father absence.

Secondly, trauma may perpetuate cycles of violence or instability, where children raised in traumatic environments are more likely to replicate these patterns in their own families. This can lead to situations where fathers feel overwhelmed or inadequate, causing them to disengage from their roles as caregivers.

Additionally, childhood trauma can create economic instability for families. Traumatized parents may have difficulty securing stable employment or managing finances, making it harder to sustain a household where both parents are present.

Overall, the complex web of emotional distress, relational challenges, and socioeconomic factors stemming from childhood trauma can result in a higher incidence of fatherless homes, perpetuating a cycle of trauma for future generations.

The absence of father figures can lead to emotional and social deficiencies in children, including feelings of abandonment and instability. According to data from the US Department of Justice, children from fatherless homes are significantly more likely to experience academic struggles, behavioral problems, and future involvement with the criminal justice system.[64] Other studies show that children from father-absent homes were more than twice as likely to be incarcerated.[65]

According to the US Census Bureau and the US Department of Justice:
- Children from fatherless homes are:

- 4 times more likely to live in poverty

- 2 times more likely to drop out of high school

- 7 times more likely to become pregnant as teenagers

- 20 times more likely to end up in prison

From the National Fatherhood Initiative's research:

- 85% of youth in prison come from fatherless homes

- Children without a father in the home are:

  - 9 times more likely to be suspended or expelled from school

  - More likely to experience behavioral problems

  - At higher risk for substance abuse

This familial disintegration can perpetuate cycles of trauma and poverty, leading to broader societal consequences such as increased reliance on social services and difficulties in community engagement.

4. Crime & Incarceration

The link between childhood trauma and criminal behavior is well-documented. Individuals who have experienced trauma may resort to crime as a maladaptive coping strategy, fueled by a need for survival or a cycle of learned behavior. High rates of incarceration strain the criminal justice system and drain public resources, while also contributing to community disintegration. Families with incarcerated members often face stigma, financial struggles, and disruption, perpetuating cycles of trauma and dysfunction.

A study published in the journal *Psychological Trauma: Theory, Research, Practice, and Policy* found that approximately 75% of male prisoners reported experiencing childhood trauma.[66] Another study found that up to 97% of juvenile offenders reported at least one adverse childhood experience, with 50% reporting four or more ACEs. This might be the source of The Compassion Project's statement that "as high as 95%" of prisoners experienced childhood trauma.[67]

5. Teen Pregnancies

Teen pregnancies are often associated with a lack of education, support, and resources, particularly among those who have experienced childhood trauma. Young parents may struggle with emotional and economic stability, frequently resulting in children who face similar adversities. High rates of teen pregnancies contribute to strained social services and educational systems, and they perpetuate cycles of poverty and instability, further fragmenting communities. Most homes of teenage pregnancies are fatherless. While specific statistics can vary, it is generally accepted that a significant majority—around 70%—of pregnancies to teenagers result in fatherless homes.

6. Sexual Molestation

Sexual molestation of a child is a devastating violation that can have profound and lasting effects on their physical, emotional, and psychological well-being. The impact varies from child to child, but common consequences include:

1. **Emotional Distress:** Children may experience feelings of confusion, shame, guilt, and fear. They often struggle with their feelings about the abuse, which can lead to anxiety, depression, and issues with self-esteem.

2. **Behavioral Changes:** A child may exhibit sudden changes in behavior, such as increased aggression, withdrawal, regression to earlier developmental stages, or acting out sexually. These behaviors can indicate their struggle to process the trauma.

3. **Trust Issues:** Victims often find it difficult to trust others, which can affect relationships with family, friends, and authority figures. This mistrust can lead to social isolation.

4. **Academic Challenges:** The emotional turmoil can impact concentration and learning, resulting in declining academic performance.

5. **Physical Symptoms:** Some children may experience unexplained physical symptoms, including changes in appetite, sleep disturbances, and psychosomatic complaints.

6. **Long-Term Effects:** The repercussions of such trauma can extend into adulthood, leading to difficulties in relationships, ongoing mental health challenges, and a higher risk of substance abuse.

The landmark ACEs study showed that women who had an early history of abuse and neglect were seven times more likely to be raped in adulthood. Women who, as children, had witnessed their mothers being assaulted by their partners had a vastly increased chance to fall victim to domestic violence.[8]

Each of these factors plays a crucial role in the disintegration of society by undermining the foundational elements of healthy relationships, economic stability, safety, and community cohesion. These challenges must be addressed collectively to rebuild and strengthen our collective societal bond.

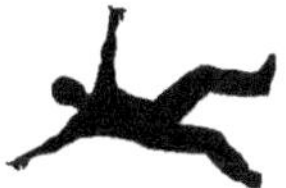

Exploring the cataclysmic societal destruction and disintegration caused by childhood trauma, it becomes painfully clear that the repercussions of early suffering stretch far beyond the individual. They weave themselves into a dark tapestry of relational dysfunction, physical health crises, spiritual disconnection, and societal decay—each thread a stark reminder of lives marred by early adversity.

The evidence laid bare throughout this chapter reveals a haunting truth: childhood trauma acts as a relentless architect of despair, erecting barriers that impede not only personal healing but also collective progress. Individuals suffer in silence, often buried beneath layers of shame, guilt, and despair, while their struggles manifest in a myriad of self-destructive behaviors, chronic illnesses, and mental health disorders. From the agonizing numbness felt by those like Camilla, to the shattered dreams of countless others forced to navigate life without a safety net of love and support, the tragedy is profound and pervasive.

While statistics indicate that nearly 70% of American adults carry the weight of childhood trauma, this is not just a data point; these numbers represent lives lost to despair, families torn apart, and communities diminished. Every single percentage point represents thousands of lives affected by ACEs. The catastrophic fallout manifests in rising rates of mental illness, substance abuse, homelessness, and even premature death.

Now we can fully understand how these devastating effects extend not only to individuals—who wrestle daily with the weight of their pain—but also to entire families, communities, and society at large. As we take stock of these outcomes, we must acknowledge the deeper implications: we are witnessing the decay of the societal fabric, a reality that extends beyond anecdotal distress into an epidemic that erodes our shared humanity.

CHAPTER FOURTEEN

The Economic Burden of Childhood Trauma

"The most dangerous phrase in the language is 'We've always done it this way.'"

–Grace Hopper

EVERY MORNING, 180 MILLION Americans wake up carrying wounds that don't just hurt their hearts—they drain the nation's wallet.[5] The child who was beaten. The teenager who was molested. The kid who watched Daddy drink himself unconscious every night. These aren't just tragic stories from the past. They're walking economic disasters, costing America more money than our entire defense budget, more than we spend on education, more than the GDP of most countries.

We've spent decades treating the symptoms while ignoring the disease. Billions pour into addiction treatment centers, mental health facilities, and prisons, yet the source of the suffering continues unchecked. We're like doctors treating fever while the patient bleeds to death internally.

The numbers are staggering. Childhood trauma costs America $14.1 trillion annually.[69] Let me repeat that: *fourteen point one trillion dollars.* To put this in perspective, that's more than the combined economic impact of cancer, heart disease, and stroke.[70] It's more than the entire GDP of China. It represents roughly 65% of America's total economic output being consumed by the aftershocks of what we do to children.

This isn't speculation or advocacy mathematics. These figures come from peer-reviewed research published in the Journal of the American Medical Association, analyzing healthcare costs, lost productivity, criminal justice expenses, social services utilization, and premature mortality across the lifespan of trauma survivors.[71]

Every single day, 1,401 Americans die from trauma-related causes.[21] Every single day. That's more than the populations of entire towns disappearing annually because of what happened to them as children. The leading cause of death in America isn't a virus or a genetic disorder—it's the accumulated damage from childhood experiences that could have been prevented.

But here's what makes this crisis particularly tragic: every dollar spent preventing childhood trauma saves $191 in lifetime costs.[72] The return on investment for trauma prevention exceeds anything Wall Street has ever produced. Yet we continue pouring money into the consequences while starving the solutions.

The individual toll is equally devastating. An adult with 4+ adverse childhood experiences will cost society $2.1 million over their lifetime in excess medical care, lost productivity, criminal justice involvement, and social services.[73] That's not the total cost of their life—that's the additional cost compared to someone who experienced a safe childhood.

This economic devastation spreads like a cancer through every sector of American society, but nowhere is it more concentrated—or more preventable—than in corporate America.

The Hidden Hemorrhage: Corporate America's Trauma Crisis

Walk into any Fortune 500 boardroom and you'll hear executives obsessing over productivity metrics, employee engagement scores, and healthcare costs. They implement wellness programs, invest in mental health benefits, and hire chief happiness officers. They speak passionately about employee well-being and corporate social responsibility.

Yet they're hemorrhaging billions to an epidemic they don't recognize, measure, or address.

I will use Johnson & Johnson as an example. J&J is the healthcare giant whose time-treated credo declares their responsibility to "doctors and nurses, to mothers and fathers and all others who use our products and services," and who employs approximately 140,000 people worldwide. Like most major corporations, J&J leadership speaks extensively about employee wellness and creating healthy workplace cultures. I know J&J truly cares for their employees, the employees' families, and the communities in which they serve.

What they don't talk about—because they are not aware—is that roughly 98,000 of their employees carry the neurobiological scars of childhood trauma.[74] These aren't weak or broken people. They're talented professionals who happen to carry invisible wounds that affect every aspect of their work performance.

The research on workplace impact is sobering. Employees with 4+ adverse childhood experiences demonstrate 280% higher rates of serious job performance problems and are 300% more likely to miss two to five additional days per month compared to their peers.[75] They exhibit significantly higher healthcare utilization, elevated rates of workplace accidents, and higher turnover requiring constant recruitment and re training.[76]

Based on established research on trauma's workplace impact, my analysis suggests Johnson & Johnson loses an estimated $944 million annually to unaddressed childhood trauma in their workforce. Nearly a billion dollars. Every single year.

This isn't money they're investing in employee development or innovative research. This is money simply evaporating due to increased absenteeism, reduced productivity, elevated healthcare costs, higher turnover, and the countless ripple effects of traumatized nervous systems trying to function in corporate environments.

The numbers across corporate America are breathtaking:

- Microsoft: $1.5 billion annually

- Morgan Stanley: $625 million annually

- Walmart: $9.2 billion annually

These aren't precise audit figures—they're my estimates based on workforce size, trauma prevalence rates, and established research on workplace impacts. But they represent a conservative calculation of costs that every major corporation faces but very few adequately measure.

The tragedy isn't just the money. It's the squandering of human potential alongside sadness and suffering. Trauma survivors face 460% higher rates of depression, 240% higher rates of chronic obstructive pulmonary disease, and are 1,132% more likely to use illegal injectable drugs.[77] Most shocking of all: employees with 6+ ACEs die an average of 20 years earlier than their colleagues.[78]

Every traumatized employee represents unrealized innovation, un-expressed leadership, undelivered excellence. Unknowingly, companies are literally paying billions for the privilege of underutilizing their own workforce.

Microsoft talks about empowering people and organizations to achieve more. Walmart emphasizes helping people save money and live better. Morgan Stanley promises to help clients achieve their financial goals while they advance economic growth worldwide. Johnson & Johnson's credo speaks of their responsibility to everyone who uses their products and services. All honest and sincere commitments.

Yet very few of these organizations—despite their stated commitments to human flourishing—have implemented comprehensive trauma-informed workplace strategies. How could they? They didn't even know. They're missing the forest for the trees, addressing symptoms while missing the root cause that's costing them billions.

But here's what should get every CEO's attention: the return on investment for trauma-informed workplace interventions is astronomical. Research indicates that trauma-informed care programs can reduce healthcare utilization by 35% and improve productivity metrics by 25%.[79] If Johnson & Johnson implemented comprehensive trauma-informed practices and improved trauma-related costs by just 20%, they would reap $188 million in annual savings. Assuming a modest implementation cost of $10 million, that's a 9,300% return on investment.

Let me say that again: *nine-thousand three-hundred percent ROI.*

Warren Buffett would mortgage his house for returns like that. Yet corporations are unknowingly walking past this opportunity every day because they don't understand the connection between childhood experiences and workplace performance. This isn't to shame and blame; these corporations' leaders just don't know.

Some forward-thinking organizations are beginning to recognize this crisis and are quietly implementing trauma-informed workplace certification. These early adopters understand that while their competitors debate wellness programs and employee satisfaction surveys, they're addressing the root cause of workplace dysfunction. They're not just gaining competitive advantages—they're building moats around their talent, creating psychologically safe environments that attract and retain the best people while dramatically reducing operational costs.

The companies that become trauma-responsive workplaces first will gain strategic advantage. Imagine the recruitment advantage when top talent sees your organization is trained to understand and address the very issues that plague 70% of the workforce. Imagine the customer loyalty when your company becomes known as an organization that truly cares about human flourishing, not just profit margins.

This isn't social work—it's a strategic business imperative. The question isn't whether corporations can afford to address childhood trauma in their workforce. The question is whether they can afford to miss the greatest competitive opportunity of the decade, and at the same time make a major contribution to improving the wellness of their employees, their families, and the community.

The blood is flowing, but the solution exists. The only question is: Which corporations will have the courage to stop treating symptoms and start healing the disease?

CHAPTER FIFTEEN

The Prevalence of Childhood Trauma

"The essence of existence eludes definition, sprawling beyond the grasp of our words, just as the depths of our unspoken sorrows shape the world we inhabit."

–Unknown

IT WAS A NIGHT filled with anticipation—the launch of my new book, attended by a vibrant crowd of 300 guests, ranging in age from 18 to 90. Among them, an equal split of men and women, all gathered to share in a moment of exploration, understanding, and hopefully, healing. As I stepped onto the stage, I felt the energy in the room, a blend of curiosity and hope. I began my speech by defining childhood trauma, a term that encompasses a spectrum of adverse experiences that can profoundly shape a child's development and lifelong health.

In an engaging attempt to connect with my audience, I asked everyone to stand. With the anticipation obvious, I then posed a simple yet profound request.

"If you have experienced childhood trauma, or if you know someone close to you who has, please take a seat."

To my astonishment, every single person sat down, immediately. In that moment, looking out at a sea of filled chairs, I felt a profound weight settle over me. That simple exercise, while unconventional, painted a stark picture: childhood trauma is a phenomenon that touches us all. I have repeated this simple survey five times now—the result is always the same.

Statistically speaking, a sample size of 300 is considered significant, and the results of my informal test were unequivocal. It confirmed my growing suspicion; that childhood trauma is not an isolated issue, it is an epidemic that affects nearly every person on this planet, manifesting in damaging ways throughout their lives. As I surveyed the room, a sobering realization hit me: the enormity of this issue transcends personal experiences and individual stories; it is a collective crisis that permeates communities and cultures globally.

The Mathematics of Universal Impact

The consistent result of my informal survey—where every person in a 300-person audience indicated they had either experienced childhood trauma or knew someone close to them who had—initially seemed remarkable. How could the reach be so universal when "only" 70% of adults report experiencing childhood trauma directly?

The answer lies in understanding how trauma ripples through families and communities, creating what I call the "mathematics of universal impact."

To illustrate this phenomenon, let's examine a theoretical corporation with 140,000 employees—similar in size to Johnson & Johnson. If we assume each employee represents a household of three people (the national average), we're looking at a total population of 420,000 individuals connected to this organization.

Using the established prevalence rate, 294,000 of these people (70%) have directly experienced childhood trauma. But the true reach extends far beyond those who experienced trauma firsthand.

The critical question becomes: In how many households does at least one person carry the burden of childhood trauma?

The mathematics reveal a startling truth. If 70% of individuals have experienced trauma, then the probability that any single person has *not* experienced trauma is 30% (0.30). In a three-person household, the probability that *all* members escaped childhood trauma is 0.30 × 0.30 × 0.30 = 0.027, or just 2.7%.

This means 97.3% of households contain at least one person who has experienced childhood trauma.

In our theoretical corporation, this translates to 408,660 people—9 7.3% of everyone connected to the organization—either experiencing trauma themselves or living with someone who has. Only 11,340 people (2.7%) exist in households completely untouched by childhood trauma.

This mathematical reality explains why childhood trauma feels omnipresent even to those who didn't experience it directly. It illuminates why my informal surveys consistently produce the same result: trauma's reach is indeed nearly universal, not because everyone experiences it personally, but because its impact radiates through every family, every workplace, every community.

The implications are profound. Childhood trauma is not a problem affecting "some people"—it is a crisis touching virtually every life in America. When we frame the issue this way, the question shifts from "Why should I care about childhood trauma?" to "How can we collectively address a crisis that affects nearly everyone we know and love?"

Prevalence is how common something is. When we talk about "the prevalence of childhood trauma," we're talking about how many children have experienced trauma—how widespread the problem really is. It's like taking a big picture view to see just how many young lives have been touched by difficult experiences, and how many carry the burden into adulthood. Think of it as counting the number of children affected by trauma out of all children in a community or country, helping us understand the true size and scope of this serious issue.

In this chapter, we will explore shocking facts and figures that highlight the pervasive nature of childhood trauma. The mere act of that audience of 300 taking their seats underscores the enormity of this issue. It is a crisis of immense proportions that cannot be overstated. Esteemed professionals such as Dr. Glenn Schiraldi, who has devoted his career to trauma healing, along with leading global experts, recognize that childhood trauma poses the most significant public health threat facing humanity today.

It is time to shed light on the profound prevalence, the sheer size of childhood trauma, in no uncertain terms. In this chapter, we will discuss the magnitude of the crisis and how we arrived at this point of destruction and disintegration. This only reinforces the urgent need for awareness, healing, and prevention.

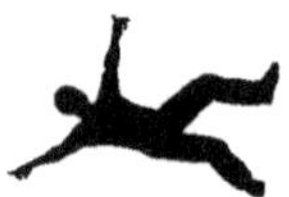

There are two landmark studies that opened our eyes and minds to the prevalence and destruction of childhood trauma: the ACEs study[8] and the Philadelphia ACEs Project.[80] The ACEs study was conducted by the Centers for Disease Control and Kaiser Permanente in the mid-1990s with a group of patients insured through Kaiser Permanente. The initial study focused on how traumatic childhood events may negatively affect adult health. The 17,421 participants surveyed were asked about their experiences with childhood neglect, abuse, family dysfunction, and current health status and behaviors.

Subsequent studies, like The Philadelphia ACE Project, have expanded the research to include data from inner-city youth, the implications of intergenerational trauma, and trauma that took place outside the home. Both studies revealed a strong correlation between childhood trauma and long-term negative health outcomes, such as increased risk for mental illness, substance abuse, and chronic physical conditions. The studies showed a direct correlation between the exposure to childhood trauma (the number of ACEs experienced) with the severity and prevalence of the disorders, illnesses, suicidality, and premature death.

Remember, in the ACEs study, an alarming 64% reported experiencing at least one ACE. The findings from the expanded ACEs study by the Philadelphia ACE Project are even more striking, with 83.2% of its 1,784 participants identifying at least one ACE in their past. The data of the prevalence of adults who experienced childhood trauma ranges from a low of 63%-83%.

So then, how many children are exposed to trauma? The natural conclusion is that 63%-83% are experiencing trauma before their eighteenth birthday, right? However, the data I can find reports a range from 14%-30%. There are several important reasons why current childhood trauma rates appear lower than adult retrospective reports.

Underreporting is likely the biggest factor explaining this discrepancy. Many cases of childhood trauma remain hidden and unreported while they're happening. Children often don't have the language, understanding, or safe opportunity to report their experiences. Parents and caregivers who are causing harm typically conceal it, and even when others suspect problems, they may hesitate to report due to uncertainty, fear of being wrong, or concerns about making things worse. Additionally, our measurement methods have improved over time, allowing us to recognize more forms of trauma than we did in the past when today's adults were children. Finally, many adults only recognize their experiences as traumatic in hindsight, after gaining perspective and understanding through maturity, therapy, or education about what constitutes trauma. What seemed "normal" to a child at the time is later understood as harmful by the adult they became.

Debating the actual size of the problem is unimportant, big is big. To err on the conservative side, I will use the lesser of the prevalence data from the two studies. I will assume for the balance of this book that 70% of all adults and children in the US have experienced childhood trauma. If you add to this those who are connected to or living with a sufferer, it is basically impacting everyone on earth. You can now understand why everyone of the 300 in the audience said they had experienced childhood trauma or knew someone who had.

Recent studies show the prevalence of childhood trauma ranges from 63-76%.[75] These results vary due to population and methodology, but tend to trend upward over time. For simplicity's sake, throughout this book, I will assume that 70% of American adults have experienced at least one adverse childhood experience.

Let's translate the percentages into numbers of people.

As I pen these words, the population of the United States stands at 332 million, comprising 258 million adults over the age of 17, and 77 million children aged 17 and younger. If we use the assumed statistic of 70% of adults who have endured childhood trauma, we arrive at a shocking reality:

180 million adults carry the heavy burden of their traumatic pasts, potentially setting the stage for life-long struggles with various disorders and illnesses and early death.

Now, let's consider the children. There are 77 million children under the age of 18 in the US, using 70%, that is 54 million young lives subjected to the horrors of trauma, their innocence shattered before they even reach adulthood. Disturbingly, many experts contend that these figures are just the tip of the iceberg, suggesting that the true numbers might be even more catastrophic. Why is this so?

The truth is, many individuals remain silent about their traumatic experiences, bound by the shackles of stigma, fear, or a simple lack of understanding about what trauma truly entails. Here is a detailed listing of the factors that I believe contribute to underreporting:

1. **Fear of Consequences:** Victims of abuse and neglect may fear retaliation from the abuser, which can include threats of further harm or abandonment. This fear can be particularly acute in cases involving family members or caregivers, leading children to remain silent about their experiences.

2. **Lack of Awareness:** Children may not recognize their experiences as abuse or neglect, especially in cases where they have grown up in environments where such behaviors are normalized. Without a clear understanding that their treatment is wrong, they may feel confused or ashamed to report it.

3. **Shame & Stigma:** Children may feel ashamed of their situation or fear judgment from peers, adults, or authorities. This shame can

discourage them from seeking help or disclosing their experiences, reinforcing the cycle of silence around trauma.

4. **Insufficient Support Systems:** Some children may lack reliable adults or supportive figures in their lives to whom they can turn for help. If they don't have a trusted adult to confide in, they are less likely to report their trauma.

5. **Cultural Factors:** Cultural norms and beliefs can influence perceptions of family privacy and the stigma surrounding reporting abuse. In some cultures, discussing family issues outside the home is discouraged, leading to underreporting.

6. **Mental Health Issues:** Childhood trauma often leads to mental health challenges such as depression, anxiety, or PTSD. These conditions can affect a child's ability to articulate their experiences, seek help, or even recognize that what they're experiencing is abuse.

7. **Inadequate Training & Resources:** Not all adults—parents, teachers, healthcare providers—are adequately trained to recognize the signs of abuse and neglect. This lack of training can mean that many cases go unnoticed or unreported even when indicators are present.

8. **Systemic Barriers:** Some families may perceive bureaucratic systems—child protective services or law enforcement—as unfriendly, unhelpful, or threatening. Experiences of systemic racism or discrimination can further discourage reporting, particularly in marginalized communities.

9. **Legal & Social Conditions:** Laws and policies surrounding mandatory reporting can vary widely and may not effectively compel reporting in all situations. Additionally, some individuals may hesitate to report for fear of legal repercussions themselves or concerns about the involvement of child protective services.

10. **Subtlety of Trauma:** Some forms of abuse and neglect can be subtle and may not leave visible marks. Emotional abuse, for instance, can

be particularly difficult to identify and report, as it may manifest in ways that are not easily recognizable or quantifiable.

So, there is reason to be confident the numbers we have do not tell the full story.

Let the numbers we *do* have sink in for a moment: 180 million adults and 54 million children, all grappling with a wide spectrum of unaddressed pain. Can you imagine any condition or disease that could be worse than childhood trauma?

Putting Real Faces on the Millions

In his best-selling book, *The Tipping Point*, Malcolm Gladwell defines the tipping point as "a place where the unexpected becomes expected, where radical change is more than a possibility. It is—contrary to all our expectations—a certainty." Writing my book, *The Kite That Couldn't Fly,* became that pivotal tipping point in my life. Initially, I set out to create a memoir for my daughters and grandchildren, but the process unfolded in ways I never could have imagined, catapulting me into the profound and often hidden world of childhood trauma.

As I dug into my own experiences and memories, I began to uncover a sobering realization: childhood trauma is not just a random personal struggle; it is an epidemic that affects millions. During the writing process and the first six months following the book's release, I was inundated with a flood of information, questions, and requests for help. Suddenly, I was confronted with real-life stories of suffering, providing tangible evidence that trauma was not an isolated occurrence but a widespread phenomenon.

My first look into the faces of this epidemic was with my own siblings. Before our discussions, all 14 of us believed we had an interesting childhood filled with some tough times, but we were completely unaware of the complex trauma that wove through our shared history. With the guidance of a few mental health professionals, we came to understand that our experiences were more than just anecdotes; they were markers of complex childhood trauma.

The consequences were haunting. Two of my brothers succumbed to drug addictions, while several of us battled depression and anxiety. Chronic health issues like heart disease, diabetes, and obesity seemed to emerge from the shadows, as if they were all part of a larger tapestry woven with trauma. Jamie, our oldest brother, finally opened up about his struggle with depression and anxiety—a battle that had silently consumed him for years. His revelation illuminated the impact of understanding and addressing trauma, significantly reshaping not only his life but also our collective consciousness as siblings.

After delving into my siblings' experiences, I found myself overwhelmed by a wave of revelations from others, each providing further evidence of what I was beginning to recognize as a widespread epidemic of childhood trauma. Friends began to share their own harrowing stories—dark memories of neglect and abuse, accompanied by the emotional scars that continued to affect their lives long after childhood had ended.

Strangers also approached me, each sharing new insights or requesting assistance. For instance, during a coffee meeting with an old friend, I discussed my writing journey on *The Kite* book. In turn, he confided in me about a deeply personal trauma. He had been sexually abused by an uncle at the age of 12, a violation that had led him to grapple with his same-sex attraction throughout his adult life, leaving him ensnared in a web of secrecy, confusion, and shame.

As our conversation concluded, a young woman named Heather, who had heard our conversation, walked up and expressed a strong interest in my book. She asked if I could notify her when it would be available. When I inquired about her interest, she shared her story of growing up in a household marked by chaos. Her mother had been married seven times before Heather turned 18, leaving her to navigate a landscape rife with dysfunction and mental health challenges. Heather was hopeful my soon-to-be published book would, in some way, help with her struggles.

On another occasion, I was shopping for a suit for an upcoming television interview about my book. I needed the suit altered by the next day, and I explained why. The salesman asked me about the book's title. As we spoke, he mentioned that he had just read a brief overview and had already ordered a copy from Amazon. Encouraged by our conversation, I gently probed him to share his own story. He revealed that he had an ACE score of 7, encompassing experiences of mental, physical, and sexual abuse. Diagnosed with four mental illnesses and three metabolic disorders, he shared how he was diligently working toward finding joy and peace in his life, making meaningful progress in his healing journey.

A significant moment occurred when the principal of an alternative high school in Philadelphia reached out to invite me to speak to 75 students. As I engaged with five different classrooms, I witnessed the profound impact of trauma on these young lives. Many of the students were teetering on the edge of the juvenile justice system or were caught up in the mental healthcare system. The staff believed that nearly all the students had faced some form of childhood trauma, with issues ranging from depression and bipolar disorder to substance abuse and violent behavior. Later that evening, I did some research and found there are approximately 10,000 such alternative schools across the US…

Case Study 6: The Alternative High School

Although not my intention, my book, *The Kite That Couldn't Fly*, quickly became a vehicle for raising awareness about the destruction caused by and the prevalence of childhood trauma. I was invited by the assistant principal to speak to the students and faculty at an alternative high school. I am confident I learned more from the students that day than they learned from me. The school enrolled 53 students aged 14 to 22 who exhibited a wide range of disorders and behaviors, including learning disabilities, addictions, mental illness, violence, and crime. Most of these students had one foot in the juvenile justice system and the other in a psychiatric ward. Many were attending the school against their will; if they did not comply, they faced incarceration.

I believed I had a good chance of connecting with the students because, in many ways, I was one of them 60 years ago. As a sophomore in high school, I was placed in an alternative school where I attended core classes in the morning and then worked as an apprentice in the afternoon. It was referred to as a "vocab school" back then, but it was also disparagingly called the program for "retards," "troubled kids," "special education," and "misfits." I could relate; I understood the shame associated with those labels.

Before speaking to the students, I had the opportunity to meet the faculty. The group was composed of impressive and dedicated teachers, social workers, and security personnel. Their mission was to help the students complete high school while teaching them essential life skills and trades with which they could support themselves. I had a few questions to help me understand the composition of the student body.

Q: What percentage of the students were taking legal medications daily?

A: 90%.

Q: What percentage of the students attended the school because of the suffering caused by childhood trauma, specifically neglect, abuse, and/or dysfunctional family dynamics?

A: Faculty responses varied, but the range was between 90% and 100%.

Q: At the last parent–teacher meeting, how many students had two loving parents in attendance who were interested in their child's progress?

A: None.

There were eight classrooms, each with between three to eight students, grouped by grade. Each class included a teacher, a social worker, and a security guard. It was not uncommon for students to need to be restrained in the classroom.

A sense of discomfort washed over me as I entered each classroom. I could instantly sense the students' anguish reflected in their reluctance to meet my gaze. The discussions we had in each classroom were rich and rewarding. Once they heard my story, they began to trust me, though they still struggled to make eye contact. By the end of the day, I spoke with one of the social workers and shared my experience of being unable to make eye contact. She quickly provided an explanation.

"The students carry strong feelings of embarrassment about their circumstances. They feel disgusted by the things they have done or that have been done to them. They cannot bear for someone like you to witness how disgraceful they think they are."

I felt a wave of sadness that tightened in my throat—the same lump that had surfaced repeatedly throughout the day.

What the social worker said made sense on the surface, but I believed there was more to this avoidance of eye contact. *Was it shame? A disorder?* That night, back in my hotel room, I googled "lack of eye contact and childhood trauma." I found a fascinating study from 2012 that compared the effects of direct eye contact on brain activation with those of an averted gaze.[81]

The study revealed a significant difference between individuals who have not experienced trauma and those who have, particularly in how their brains respond to eye contact. Normally, the prefrontal cortex—the area of the brain that helps us think, assess others, and understand their intentions—activates when we see someone approaching. However, individuals who have experienced trauma show minimal to no activity in this region, indicating they struggle to feel curiosity about others.

This means that when someone who has experienced childhood trauma is looked at directly, they may enter survival mode rather than engage.

What does this imply for their ability to form friendships and interact with others? It raises questions about their capacity to trust anyone with their fears. Building genuine relationships requires seeing others as individuals with their own thoughts and reasons. However, people who have faced trauma may have difficulty understanding this concept and may struggle to assert themselves. This confusion can lead to poor decision-making, rendering them easy targets for exploitation.

It is a well-documented fact that individuals who experience trauma in childhood face a dramatically increased risk of developing addictions, becoming victims of sexual assault as adults, experiencing teenage pregnancy, and committing crimes. Is it possible that the compromise of the prefrontal cortex caused by childhood trauma is partly or wholly to blame? Predators can sense this neurological vulnerability like sharks detect blood in water, seeking out those whose brain's defense systems have been weakened—as my friend Sarah witnessed firsthand among traumatized children in Amazonia.

Another poignant encounter took place while I was discussing my book with a web designer over the phone. As I explained the book's purpose, he broke down in tears, revealing that his 12-year-old sister had recently taken her own life. He shared that she had been sexually molested by a family member, and the weight of this trauma had become unbearable for her. In his grief, he offered to volunteer his services, wanting to contribute in any way he could to support the cause.

My most memorable face of trauma came when I was introduced to Trent, a friend of a friend who had read my book.

Case Study 7: Trent's Journey

Trent was the epitome of success, a shining example of the American dream realized. By all outward measures, he seemed to have it all: a devoted wife, two loving children, and a flourishing career that took him from a humble beginning folding clean towels at a local car wash to becoming a multimillionaire by age 40. His energy, creativity, and tenacity propelled him to the forefront of multiple businesses in the auto industry, earning him the admiration of peers and the respect of his family. After a lifetime of hard work, he made the decision to retire at age 50, ready to relish in the fruits of his labor.

However, just weeks after stepping away from his career, everything began to unravel. What started as moments of unease quickly spiraled into overwhelming despair. Trent's mind became a battleground filled with intrusive thoughts, culminating in the harrowing contemplation of suicide. He found himself in a desperate darkness, feeling as if he was losing his grip on reality.

Trent described what he was experiencing as a force that pulled him to the ground. At times, he said he found it difficult to even move his body. During one of our talks, he whispered hopelessly, "It's a force greater than gravity." Getting to know Trent was a tipping point in my journey. It was his story that initiated the writing of this book and selecting its title, *Greater Than Gravity*.

In a moment of crisis, he crashed his car into a tree, leading to a series of hospital visits that saw him in and out of psychiatric wards. Each doctor he encountered offered a different diagnosis, but none could provide him the clarity he desperately sought.

Questions about his childhood began to stir within him, yet clarity eluded him. His first tangible memory was of being placed in a program for troubled children at Duke University when he was just a boy. Driven by a need for answers, Trent sought out his hospital records from that time. What he discovered was chilling. He was admitted at the behest of his mother, who had claimed he attempted to kill his younger sister with a baseball bat. The story haunted him but lacked context.

Fueled by a deep sense of betrayal, Trent confronted his mother, seeking the truth behind the painful memories that danced just beyond the reach of his recollection. The moment was a watershed for both mother and son; as she broke down, the barriers of silence and shame shattered. She confessed the truth, revealing that he had never tried to kill his sister. Instead, she had fabricated the story to have him removed from the home, claiming he was "difficult."

What she shared next opened the door for Trent's quest for healing and understanding: from the age of just six weeks old, she had been beating him with a wooden spoon two to three times a day, continuing this pattern for the first four years of his life. Eventually, Trent's father also took part, subjecting him to physical discipline for a variety of inappropriate and unfair reasons.

This revelation, though harrowing, became pivotal in Trent's journey toward healing. Armed with a new understanding of his past, he began to connect the dots between the trauma of his childhood and the struggles he faced in adulthood. Recognizing that the profound impact of early life experiences could resurface even decades later was the first step toward reclaiming his narrative. Determined to find sanity and reclaim joy, Trent embarked on a journey of therapy, reflection, and personal growth. He began to unpack the layers of his childhood trauma, transforming his pain into a narrative of survival and resilience.

Through relentless work, both on himself and with professional guidance, Trent slowly learned to confront the shadows of his past. He not only sought to understand his mother's actions but also to forgive his own experiences, recognizing that healing does not mean forgetting. His transformation inspired not just his family but also countless others, proving that even the most seemingly successful lives can bear hidden wounds that, when acknowledged, pave the way for renewed hope and vitality.

Each interaction surrounding this topic has deepened my understanding of the pervasive nature of childhood trauma, reinforcing my resolve to shed light on this crucial issue through the writing of this book, *Greater Than Gravity*.

Research by the Centers for Disease Control and Prevention has shown that one in five Americans was sexually molested as a child; one in four was beaten by a parent to the point of a mark being left on their body; and one in three couples engages in physical violence. A quarter of us grew up with alcoholic relatives, and one out of eight witnessed their mother being beaten or hit.[3, 17]

Trauma happens to so many of us, our friends, our families, and our neighbors.

CHAPTER SIXTEEN

The Hidden Epidemic

Revealing Childhood Trauma's True Burden Through Advanced Epidemiological Analysis

"It's time we begin viewing childhood trauma as the highly contagious, life-threatening disease that it is. By all measures, childhood trauma is an epidemic."

–Michael Menard

The Methodological Blind Spot

FOR DECADES, EPIDEMIOLOGISTS HAVE employed a fundamentally flawed approach to measuring disease burden that systematically underestimates the most devastating health threats of our time. Our current mortality tracking system—focused on proximate causes recorded on death certificates—captures only the final medical event while ignoring the upstream factors that set individuals on pathways to premature death decades earlier.

This methodological limitation has created a massive blind spot in public health understanding, leading us to fight symptoms while ignoring root causes, allocate resources based on incomplete data, and miss opportunities for the most impactful interventions possible. Nowhere is this more evident than in our failure to recognize childhood trauma's true epidemiological burden.

The time has come for a methodological revolution in how we measure, understand, and respond to the greatest threats to human flourishing.

The Current System's Fatal Flaw

"The most dangerous phrase in the language is, 'We've always done it this way.'"

–Grace Hopper

Traditional epidemiological approaches suffer from what I call "medical event myopia"—the tendency to focus exclusively on the immediate cause of death while ignoring the complex causal chain of events that led to that moment. When a 45-year-old dies of a heart attack, current methodology records "cardiovascular disease." When a 25-year-old commits suicide, we record "intentional self-harm." When a 35-year-old dies of an overdose, we blame "accidental poisoning."

But what if the heart attack resulted from 30 years of chronic stress, smoking, and metabolic dysfunction triggered by childhood sexual abuse? What if the suicide followed decades of depression and PTSD stemming from severe neglect? What if the overdose represented the final stage of addiction that began as a teenager's attempt to numb the pain of repeated violence?

Our current system would classify these as three separate medical events with no connection to their common origin: childhood trauma. This is not just an academic distinction—it represents a fundamental misunderstanding of disease causation that has profound implications for prevention, treatment, and resource allocation.

The Established Precedent for Root-Cause Attribution

The epidemiological community has already recognized this limitation in certain contexts and developed sophisticated methodologies to address it. The most successful example is tobacco-related mortality. When a lifelong smoker dies of lung cancer, epidemiologists correctly attribute that death to smoking, not merely to "respiratory failure" or "malignant neoplasm."

This attribution relies on Population Attributable Fraction (PAF) methodology, which calculates the proportion of disease burden attributable to specific risk factors based on their prevalence in the population and their relative risk of causing adverse outcomes. Using this approach, researchers have demonstrated that tobacco kills approximately 480,000 Americans annually—deaths that would be invisible if we relied solely on immediate causes listed on death certificates.

The success of attribution methodology provides both scientific precedent and methodological framework for applying similar analysis to other upstream risk factors. The question is not whether such analysis is scientifically valid—it's why we haven't applied it systematically to childhood trauma.

The Childhood Trauma Evidence Base

The epidemiological evidence linking childhood trauma to premature mortality is overwhelming and continues to grow. A meta-analysis of the landmark Adverse Childhood Experiences (ACEs) study, involving over 17,421 participants, demonstrated dose-response relationships between childhood trauma exposure and leading causes of death in adulthood.[49]

Subsequent research has expanded and refined these findings across diverse populations. A comprehensive meta-analysis of thirty studies involving over 250,000 participants found that childhood trauma exposure increases mortality risk by 45% on average, with some forms of trauma doubling or tripling lifetime mortality risk.[15] These effects persist after controlling for socioeconomic status, education, and other potential confounding variables.

The biological mechanisms underlying these associations are increasingly well-understood. Childhood trauma triggers chronic activation of stress response systems, leading to dysregulation of the hypothalamic-pituitary-adrenal axis, persistent inflammation, the destruction of mitochondria, accelerated cellular aging, and epigenetic changes that increase vulnerability to physical and mental health problems throughout life.[19] This "biological embedding" of early adversity provides the physiological pathway from childhood trauma to premature death years and even decades later.

Years of Life Lost: A Superior Metric

Traditional mortality statistics suffer from another critical limitation: they treat all deaths as equivalent. A death certificate approach gives equal weight to an 85-year-old cancer patient who dies three years before statistical life expectancy and a 25-year-old trauma survivor who completes suicide, losing 55 potential years of life.

Years of Life Lost (YLL) methodology addresses this limitation by weighting deaths according to the years of life cut short by premature mortality. This approach has gained widespread acceptance in epidemiology and health policy because it better captures the true societal burden of different health conditions.[82]

When we apply YLL analysis to childhood trauma, its devastating impact becomes immediately apparent. Trauma-related deaths occur disproportionately among younger populations—through suicide, overdose, violence, and stress-accelerated chronic disease. This age distribution creates enormous YLL totals that dwarf all other leading causes of mortality.

Consider the epidemiological reality: While cancer and heart disease primarily kill older adults with limited remaining life expectancy, childhood trauma kills people across the entire age spectrum, with particularly high mortality rates among adolescents and young adults. A single trauma-related suicide at age 25 represents more years of life lost than multiple cancer deaths among elderly patients.

The Staggering Revelation: 1.783 Billion Years Stolen

Using precise data from foundational epidemiological studies, I have calculated what no researcher has ever quantified: the total Years of Life Lost to childhood trauma in America.[83] The results should shock the nation to its core.

Childhood trauma will steal 1.783 BILLION years of life from Americans.

One billion seven-hundred eighty-three million years. This represents more than 23 million complete human lifespans—an entire phantom nation worth of years, simply vanish into the void of preventable, premature death.

I do not yet have reliable data to calculate the global toll, but I will estimate it at upwards of 40 billion years lost, solely by extrapolating US data.

The Calculation That Changes Everything:

My analysis of foundational ACE study data reveals the precise dose-response relationship between childhood trauma exposure and premature mortality:

- 1 ACE exposure: 2 years of life lost on average

- 2 ACEs: 4 years of life lost

- 3 ACEs: 6 years of life lost

- 4 ACEs: 8 years of life lost

- 6+ ACEs: 20 years of life lost[2]

When applied to current US population data showing ACE prevalence by exposure level, the cumulative devastation becomes clear: **1.783 billion years of human life will be stolen by preventable childhood trauma.**

To grasp this astronomical theft:

- This equals the combined lifespans of everyone in California, Texas, Florida, and New York

- It represents more years than all of recorded human civilization since ancient Egypt

- It's equivalent to losing 127,000 years of human life *every single day*

- Childhood trauma steals more than 88 complete lifetimes every hour

The Comparison That Should End All Debate

While America mobilizes hundreds of billions of dollars to fight other diseases, Years of Life Lost analysis reveals our catastrophically misguided priorities:

Total Years of Life Lost in America:
- Childhood Trauma: 1.783 BILLION years stolen

- Cancer: 8.7 million years lost

- Heart Disease: 7.2 million years lost

- Stroke: 1.3 million years lost

- All Accidents Combined: 5.1 million years lost

- COVID-19 (peak year): 9.6 million years lost[82]

Childhood trauma steals more years of American life than cancer, heart disease, stroke, accidents, and COVID-19 combined—multiplied by 195.

We spend more than $200 billion annually fighting cancer that steals 8.7 million years. We spent trillions fighting COVID-19 that stole 9.6 million years at its peak. Yet we virtually ignore the condition stealing 1.783 billion years—more than 200 times the devastation of diseases that dominate our national health agenda.

The Human Reality Behind the Numbers

These 1.783 billion stolen years represent real human experiences:

- 1.783 billion Christmas mornings that will never happen

- 1.783 billion years of grandchildren who will never be held

- 1.783 billion years of innovations never created

- 1.783 billion years of love never given

- 1.783 billion years of wisdom never shared

This is your neighbor dying at 45 from trauma-induced heart disease, losing 35 years with family. Your coworker's daughter completing suicide at 22, eliminating 58 years of potential. Entire communities trapped in cycles of early death that rob them of their elders, wisdom-keepers, and experienced leaders.

The Corporate Recognition Gap

The corporate world's blindness to this epidemic is just as staggering. In a hypothetical 140,000-employee workforce:

Years of Life Lost:

- Childhood trauma: 968,000 years stolen from workers

- Cancer: 48 million years lost

- Heart disease: 26 million years lost

- All other diseases combined: <200 million years lost

Childhood trauma steals six times more years from American workers than every other disease combined.

Yet corporate wellness programs spend billions screening for cancer and heart disease while ignoring the vastly more destructive epidemic operating in 70% of cubicles, offices, and boardrooms.

The Economic Magnitude of Misallocation

Our methodological blind spot has created massive misallocations of healthcare resources and research funding. The National Cancer Institute receives approximately $6.9 billion annually in federal funding, supporting research into diseases that result in 8.7 million years of life lost. Meanwhile, childhood trauma research—addressing conditions that will cause 1.783 billion years of life lost—receives a fraction of comparable investment.

This resource misallocation extends throughout the healthcare system. Billions are spent on cardiac interventions, cancer treatments, and other downstream medical interventions that address symptoms of trauma-related pathology while virtually ignoring the upstream prevention and treatment of trauma itself.

When childhood trauma shortens lives by decades rather than years, the economic impact compounds exponentially. Each of those 1.783 billion to be stolen years represents lost productivity, reduced tax revenue, increased social service costs, and immeasurable human capital destruction.

The Path Forward: Methodological Innovation

Addressing this epidemiological blind spot requires systematic methodological innovations across multiple domains:

Enhanced Mortality Attribution: Death certificate systems should incorporate upstream risk factor attribution, like tobacco-related mortality tracking. This requires training medical examiners and coroners to identify and record trauma histories when relevant to cause of death.

Population Health Surveillance: Public health surveillance systems should routinely collect and analyze trauma exposure data alongside traditional disease monitoring. The Behavioral Risk Factor Surveillance System's ACE module provides a foundation, but expanded implementation is needed.

Years of Life Lost Emphasis: YLL should become a primary metric for health burden assessment, resource allocation, and prevention priority-setting. This shift would immediately highlight conditions like childhood trauma that disproportionately affect younger populations.

Research Funding Realignment: Federal research funding should be allocated proportional to true disease burden as measured by YLL. This would dramatically increase investment in childhood trauma prevention and treatment research proportional to its 1.783 billion years of annual impact.

The Urgent Imperative

The epidemiological evidence is clear: Childhood trauma represents the most devastating threat to population health in modern society. Its 1.783 billion years of annual life theft extends far beyond traditional health metrics, affecting educational attainment, economic productivity, criminal justice involvement, and intergenerational transmission of adversity.

Yet our current epidemiological framework systematically obscures this impact, creating a dangerous illusion that we understand our most pressing health challenges. We spend billions fighting downstream symptoms while the upstream cause continues stealing 127,000 years of life daily.

The cost of this methodological blind spot is measured not just in research dollars misallocated or prevention programs underfunded, but in 1.783 billion years of human potential vanishing annually into preventable, premature death.

The Greater Than Gravity Revelation

Childhood trauma operates like an invisible force pulling down human potential across all levels of society. Like gravity, it affects nearly everyone (70% of adults experienced at least one adverse childhood experience[8]), remains largely invisible until measured, shapes life trajectories from the moment of impact, compounds its effects over time, and cannot be ignored or wished away.

This "trauma gravity" explains patterns of dysfunction, disease, and premature death that have puzzled epidemiologists for decades. The 1.783 billion years it will steal represents the inexorable pull of untreated childhood wounds on human civilization itself.

Understanding trauma as this gravitational force should transform our approach to public health intervention. Rather than fighting individual symptoms as they emerge, we can address the fundamental force creating those symptoms. Rather than accepting certain populations' poor health outcomes as inevitable, we can intervene at the source of their trajectory alteration.

The epidemiological revolution has begun. The question is whether we will lead it or be overwhelmed by the continued devastation of 1.783 billion years of preventable trauma–related life theft annually. The choice—and the opportunity—is ours.

Let's take a look at a few groups that include millions of people in the US alone that are impacted by childhood trauma.

Those With Depression

In October of 2023 the National Institute of Mental Health (NIMH) reported there are 21 million cases of depression in the US. As we discussed earlier, the number is most likely higher due to logical rationale for underreporting. And of the 21 million, the Centers for Disease Control and Prevention (CDC) reports that 44% of all depression cases, that's a group of 9.2 million, suffer from depression caused by their exposure to childhood trauma.

Low Income Families

As we look into the complex relationship between low-income status and the prevalence of ACEs, I want to emphasize a critical point: childhood trauma is not exclusive to the impoverished. It is a pervasive issue that transcends socioeconomic barriers, affecting children from all backgrounds. While it is essential to highlight the heightened risk of ACEs faced by low-income children, it is just as important to avoid perpetuating stigma or the misconception that childhood trauma is solely a problem for the poor.

The original ACEs study from 1995, which involved 17,421 participants of which 80% were from white, middle-class backgrounds, revealed a significant prevalence of childhood trauma—64%. This foundational research demonstrated that trauma can and does occur across various socioeconomic groups. However, it was the 2017 Philadelphia study that expanded our understanding of ACEs in a broader context, incorporating a more diverse group of participants, many of whom came from inner city, low-income areas. This study reported an alarming prevalence rate of 83%, particularly when accounting for the impact of community violence and other environmental stressors prevalent in under-resourced neighborhoods not included in the original ACEs study.

There is a well-documented correlation between low income and childhood trauma. Children from low-income families are disproportionately affected by ACEs, which include abuse, neglect, domestic violence, community violence, food insecurity, and parental substance abuse. The stresses associated with poverty, such as financial instability, lack of access to healthcare, inadequate housing conditions, and limited educational opportunities, exacerbate the risks of trauma, creating a cascade of challenges that many low-income children must navigate.

In the US, approximately 15 million children live in families with incomes below the federal poverty line. These children are at greater risk for experiencing various forms of trauma. Research reveals that socioeconomic status can significantly influence a child's experience of ACEs; studies show that children from low-income backgrounds are more likely to encounter multiple ACEs compared to their higher-income counterparts. For instance, a report published by the Centers for Disease Control and Prevention (CDC) indicates that children living in poverty are nearly twice as likely to experience two or more ACEs than those from higher-income families. The original ACEs studies also reveal that if a child experiences just one ACE, they are 87% more likely to be exposed to additional ACEs.

By exploring the intersection of poverty and childhood trauma, we can hopefully foster a more nuanced understanding that respects the shared experiences of all children while simultaneously addressing the specific systemic issues that disproportionately impact those in low-income communities. I approach this with the intent to educate, uplift, and advocate for a comprehensive understanding of childhood trauma as a multi-dimensional issue.

The implications of these experiences are profoundly concerning. Childhood trauma can lead to long-term physical and mental health issues, affecting academic performance and future employability. For example, children exposed to multiple ACEs are at a heightened risk for developing mental health disorders, such as anxiety and depression. If they do experience mental disorders of any kind, pathways open to develop chronic, metabolic health conditions later in life. Furthermore, children from low-income families often lack access to supportive resources, such as mental health services and nurturing environments, further compounding the effects of trauma and limiting their opportunities for recovery and growth.

To address this pressing issue, targeted interventions and policy changes are crucial. Programs that offer mental health support, educational resources, and community-based assistance can help mitigate the impact of trauma on low-income children. Additionally, promoting economic stability through job training, affordable housing, and social services can create a more supportive environment for families, reducing the risk of childhood trauma.

Fatherless Homes

A staggering 8.3 million children in the US live in fatherless homes, a situation that significantly heightens their risk of experiencing childhood trauma. While there are, of course, single mothers doing a beautiful job raising and caring for their children, the absence of a father figure often contributes to instability, emotional distress, and a lack of support. This absence can lead to heightened vulnerability to a range of adverse experiences, including but not limited to neglect, abuse, and exposure to community violence.

Research indicates that children in fatherless homes are at a disproportionately higher risk of experiencing emotional and behavioral issues. A study revealed that children without an involved father show more significant signs of anxiety, depression, and aggression compared to their peers living in two-parent households.[84] The emotional void created by the absence of a father figure can hinder a child's social development, leading to difficulties in forming healthy relationships, managing stress, and regulating emotions.[85]

Additionally, children in fatherless homes are more likely to encounter economic hardships, further exacerbating their vulnerability to childhood trauma. They often live in single-parent households that face financial challenges, which can create an environment filled with stress and instability. Poverty itself is a well-established risk factor for trauma, and when combined with the absence of a father, this dynamic can lead to a perfect storm of adverse experiences. For instance, researchers have found that children living in poverty are more likely to experience neglect and abuse, with many studies indicating higher rates of all forms of maltreatment in households without fathers.

The correlation between fatherlessness and negative adult outcomes is also well documented. Adults who experienced parental absence during childhood often report higher levels of mental health issues, such as depression and anxiety. Moreover, studies have indicated that individuals from fatherless homes may face difficulties in achieving academic success, stable employment, and healthy relationships as adults. The National Fatherhood Initiative notes that children from fatherless homes are more likely to encounter behavioral problems, substance abuse, and criminal activity, perpetuating cycles of trauma and instability.[86] Another study found that boys who grew up in father-absent homes were significantly more likely to be incarcerated than those from two-parent homes, highlighting the potential for intergenerational cycles of family disruption and criminal behavior.[65]

Furthermore, the absence of a father figure can detrimentally impact a child's self-esteem and sense of identity. The formation of a positive self-concept is instrumental in navigating life's challenges, and children who grow up without an engaged father may struggle with feelings of inadequacy or worthlessness. Such emotional scars can influence how they perceive themselves in adulthood, affecting their relationships, career choices, and overall quality of life.

Despite these challenges, it is crucial to recognize that not all children from fatherless homes are destined to experience negative outcomes.

Many single mothers and guardians provide robust emotional support and nurturing environments that foster resilience. Targeted interventions, such as mentorship programs, community support systems, and access to mental health resources can play a pivotal role in breaking the cycle of trauma and promoting positive development.

The correlation between childhood trauma and fatherlessness is multifaceted and it demands our attention. We must learn more and do more. While the absence of a father figure may contribute significantly to emotional and behavioral challenges during childhood, and affect outcomes in adulthood, it is imperative to approach this topic with sensitivity and an understanding of the diverse experiences and strengths of families. Implementing effective education, support systems, and interventions can empower these children to navigate their circumstances and build healthier futures.

A God-Sized Problem

As we shift our focus from the troubling prevalence of childhood trauma in America to a broader perspective, it becomes increasingly evident that this crisis knows no borders. The profound impact of childhood trauma extends far beyond the confines of urban neighborhoods and suburban homes; it is a global epidemic affecting children from all walks of life. From the bustling streets of Philadelphia to remote villages in the Amazon, the circumstances may differ, but the underlying challenges resonate with alarming consistency.

I found limited data on the global prevalence of childhood trauma, which illustrates the severe lack of research conducted on the issue at that scale. The information I did discover from the World Health Organization is striking: an estimated one billion children worldwide experience trauma *each year* due to neglect, abuse, and dysfunctional households.[87,88] These traumatic experiences significantly shape their development and future potential. If we apply the conservative estimate of 70% prevalence in adults in the United States, as discussed earlier, that translates to approximately 3.5 billion individuals who have faced childhood trauma globally. This incomprehensible estimation underscores an urgent need for increased awareness, intervention, and support across the globe.

I attended a fundraiser for Justice & Mercy International (JMI) in Nashville, Tennessee. The organization is dedicated to preventing human trafficking and providing care for vulnerable children, among other developmental initiatives. Sarah, the director of JMI for the Amazonia region of Brazil, took the stage to share the impactful work she and her team are doing with the donations.

With a heavy heart, Sarah spoke about the alarming prevalence of human trafficking and child abuse in the tribes and communities throughout Amazonia. One particularly harrowing aspect she addressed was the epidemic of sexual abuse among the very young girls, specifically highlighting the tragic occurrence of incest. She recounted her conversations with a local elder about the destructive consequences of such abuse and his chilling remark. "Take my twelve-year-old granddaughter. Someone must be her first; why shouldn't it be me?"

In that moment, Sarah conveyed the profound urgency she felt, sharing that she had heard a powerful message from God: "Enough, this must stop now!" Her words resonated deeply with everyone in attendance, amplifying the need for immediate action to protect vulnerable children in the region and further convincing me that childhood trauma is a global crisis.

The Kite That Couldn't Fly had barely been on the shelves for a month when a mysterious email from Dr. Lee Long landed in my inbox, bearing the subject line "A World Changing Dinner." Dr. Long is the founder of Restoration Counseling, a renowned organization devoted to healing trauma. Intrigued yet apprehensive, I accepted the invitation, unaware of the life-altering revelations that awaited me.

The evening arrived, and I found myself seated at an elegantly set table with five unfamiliar faces. As we each introduced ourselves, a peculiar thread wove through our introductions. One by one, we concluded with the same confounding confession, "I have no idea why I am here, but I am grateful for the invitation and eager to discover our purpose." It was strange, but I couldn't shake the feeling that each of us had been pulled to this gathering for a reason far beyond mere coincidence.

The last to speak was Eric Watt, the founder of Reaching Unreachable Nations (RUN). His credentials were impressive; RUN has planted over three million Christian home churches and is at the forefront of the battle against human trafficking across continents—Africa, Asia, and Europe, including the Middle East. But it was his words about the children they rescue that set my heart racing. Eric painted a haunting picture of vulnerable children, victims of tragedy and trauma, bearing the weight of unthinkable abuse. With urgency in his voice, he revealed that RUN had salvaged over 630,000 children from the grips of despair, placing them in nurturing foster church homes whenever possible.

His words crystallized the truth around us. We weren't just strangers brought together by fate; we were gathered to confront a shared burden: the healing of those 630,000 children who were desperately seeking a way back to innocence. Eric's eyes gleamed with passion as he shared his hope that, together, we could find transformative solutions for their suffering.

I sat frozen, acutely aware of my place in the room. I was simply an author who had penned a memoir about my own turbulent childhood.

I felt the piercing weight of doubt; I belonged here, yet I didn't. I had no expertise in healing wounds or fighting such widespread despair.

"I think you have the wrong person," I ventured gently. "I really don't know how I can help."

Eric wasn't swayed. He leaned in, his conviction unyielding.

"This is a God-sized problem that demands a God-sized solution." His voice echoed with a power that seemed to fill the room. He reminded me of the miracles of old—how the God who parted the Red Sea for the Israelites still moves in ways we can scarcely comprehend. Then, he revealed he had read my book about kites, and he believed it was a steppingstone toward ending the cycle of childhood trauma.

In that moment, something shifted within me. The urgency of the task at hand began to outweigh my self-doubt. With a mix of resolve and trepidation, I found myself responding with two simple words.

"I'm in."

As the dinner drew to a close, I couldn't shake the weight of this insidious reality. Every child lost to trauma is more than just a statistic; their stories are woven into the fabric of a global epidemic, affecting literally billions around the world. This dinner was a solemn reminder: childhood trauma knows no borders and demands our collective action.

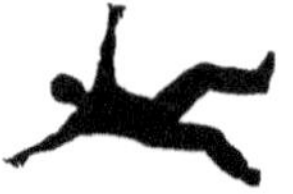

As we zoom in on the intimate experiences of my siblings and simultaneously pull back to examine the broader global landscape, we confront a chilling reality: we are in the midst of a silent pandemic—a pandemic of childhood trauma that is quietly yet insidiously impacting humanity as a whole.

This book serves as a snapshot of our current state in 2025—a reflection of the "What is." And the truth of that reality is unsettling. But as I ponder this question—are we moving toward healing, or are we careening toward catastrophe? —I can't shake the feeling that we are teetering on the edge of a deeper crisis.

Obsessed with the trajectory of this unseen contagion, I find myself grappling with a single, stark dot of data. We stand in a realm devoid of clear trends, where the absence of upward or downward movement leaves us suspended in uncertainty. My assumption—whether right or wrong—is daunting: approximately 70% of our population continues to wrestle with the scars of childhood trauma. While there are noble movements, extensive research, and impactful projects aimed at fostering awareness and spearheading interventions, we must confront a sobering truth: these efforts are merely scratching the surface of a colossal problem.

Without a robust historical context and a reliable lens through which to forecast our future, we are left navigating in the dark. Yet, we possess the power to envision what lies ahead, to influence our trajectory, and to create plausible futures. The questions we must ask ourselves become imperative if we are ever to construct the solutions necessary to dismantle this pandemic.

Despite the lack of solid data, an unsettling hypothesis has taken root within me—one that shifts from hope to dread. My instinct is that the fallout from childhood trauma is on the verge of escalating into something far worse. As the echoes of the COVID-19 pandemic continue to reverberate through our lives, its implications for the mental and emotional well-being of our children loom. Are we truly prepared for the storm that may be brewing on the horizon?

A New Kind of Generational Trauma

As the world grappled with the COVID-19 pandemic in 2020, a myriad of protective measures were swiftly implemented with the belief they would curb the virus's spread. The pandemic and subsequent protection measures introduced numerous other challenges that posed significant risks to children's development, particularly during their formative years. I am concerned that we will see the ramifications of this international, traumatic external event as those who were children in 2020 become adults.

The following are four other potential threats to children's development attributed to COVID-19:

Social Isolation: Lockdowns, social distancing mandates, and the closure of schools and recreational activities have resulted in prolonged periods of isolation for many children. This lack of social interaction can hinder the development of essential social skills, such as empathy, communication, and conflict resolution. Prolonged isolation can also exacerbate feelings of loneliness and anxiety, leading to potential long-term emotional and mental health issues.

Disruption of Education: The abrupt transition to remote learning presented significant challenges for children, especially for those from disadvantaged backgrounds or with learning disabilities. The lack of in-person instruction can lead to educational gaps and developmental delays, particularly in foundational skills such as literacy and numeracy. The uncertainty surrounding schooling may further contribute to increased anxiety among children concerning their education and future prospects.

Increased Household Stress: The pandemic has placed considerable strain on families, resulting in heightened stress levels within households. Factors such as job loss, financial insecurity, and health concerns can create a toxic environment that adversely affects children's emotional well-being. Children in high-stress environments may experience increased anxiety, disruptive behaviors, and challenges in emotional regulation, which can hinder their overall development and attachment to caregivers.

Interruption of Developmentally Critical Attachment: Evidence shows that newborns rely heavily on an array of social cues, particularly facial expressions, to form attachments and understand emotional signals. The protective bond between an infant and its primary caregiver is perhaps the most crucial relationship in human development. It is during these formative years that a child learns to navigate the world, emulating behavior, sensing safety, and developing trust.

Research has demonstrated that when infants are deprived of seeing their mother's face, or seeing an unhappy face, it can trigger stress responses that lead to significant physiological changes. When a mother's face is masked, the critical comforting signals—the warmth of a smile, the reassurance of eye contact—are effectively dampened. The resulting stress hormones that flood a child's developing brain can distort neural pathways essential for emotional regulation, social interactions, and overall mental health.

The potential explosion of childhood trauma in the wake of the COVID-19 pandemic is very real. As we discussed in chapters 9 and 10, childhood trauma often translates into mental and physical disorders and illnesses later in life. The pandemic of childhood trauma is not just a fleeting consequence of an unprecedented time; it is just possibly a ticking time bomb that demands our attention and action. What may have been necessary measures for immediate health could also constitute an unintentional yet far-reaching force, setting in motion a cascade of effects that could reverberate for years to come. If we are to halt the train of generational trauma, we must act with urgency and intention, and turn our collective gaze toward healing and restoration.

The reality is that childhood trauma itself is a tangible contagion, one that affects nearly every person on Earth, overshadowing the impacts of heart disease, cancer, stroke, and diabetes *combined.* With an estimated 3.5 billion people globally burdened by this unseen epidemic, this is clearly a systemic health crisis demanding immediate attention and collective action. In a world where childhood trauma is often hidden in the shadows, we are confronted with a profound truth: it is a global epidemic that carries both emotional and physical consequences for hundreds of millions, maybe even billions, influencing mental health, longevity, and societal stability.

This clarion call for awareness, intervention, and healing challenges us to confront the pervasive yet seldom-acknowledged toll of childhood trauma on humanity.

Soon, you will discover my personal perspective on what I believe needs to happen to turn the tide on this dreadful aspect of humanity. But before we can forge a path toward meaningful solutions and effective interventions, we must first turn our gaze inward and examine the roots of this pervasive issue. Understanding how we arrived at this point in society allows us to unravel the intricate web of factors that contribute to the epidemic of childhood trauma.

CHAPTER SEVENTEEN

Love Wasn't Enough

"It is easier to build strong children than to repair broken men."

–Frederick Douglass

LET ME TELL YOU about a child I'll call Darius.

By age seven, Darius had lived in four different homes. By twelve, the count was nine. Each time a placement failed, his file grew thicker with notes about his "behavioral problems"—the aggression, the lying, the hoarding of food under his mattress, the way he flinched when adults moved too quickly.

His foster parents tried. God knows they tried. But nothing in the standard foster parent training prepared them for a child who couldn't make eye contact because eye contact once meant danger. Nothing explained why he raged when asked about his day at school—because in his previous home, that question preceded beatings. Nothing taught them that his brain had been literally rewired by years of chaos and fear, that his nervous system was stuck in survival mode, scanning for threats that no longer existed but that his body couldn't forget.

One by one, his foster families gave up. Not because they didn't care. Because they weren't equipped. They were given a traumatized child and told to love him. Love wasn't enough.

Darius aged out of the system at eighteen. Within two years, he was homeless. Within three, incarcerated. His story is a tragedy. It is also a statistic—one that repeats itself hundreds of thousands of times across America every year.

The Scope of the Crisis

As of the most recent federal estimates, there are more than 400,000 children in the foster care system in the United States at any given time.[89] Every single one of them has experienced adverse childhood experiences—abuse, neglect, or familial instability severe enough to warrant removal from their home. These early traumas have profound effects on their emotional and psychological well-being, leading to higher rates of mental health issues, educational challenges, and difficulty forming stable relationships as they grow older.

But here is the number that should keep every policymaker, every pastor, every citizen awake at night: **seventy to eighty percent of youth who age out of the foster care system will face homelessness, addiction, imprisonment, or trafficking within three years.**[90]

Read that again. Seven or eight out of every ten children we are supposed to be protecting will, by age twenty-one, end up on the streets, in prison, addicted, or exploited.

Nationally, more than 20,000 young people age out of the foster care system every year without being placed with a permanent family.[89] Research indicates that approximately twenty percent of former foster youth become homeless within just a few years of aging out. Nearly half of young adults who have been in foster care report struggling with unemployment and mental health challenges.[90]

The consequences are staggering. With the assumption that foster children will experience an average of four or more ACEs before they turn eighteen, predictions based on the ACEs study reveal a devastating future for these individuals. Sixty thousand of them will die 25 years earlier than their peers who have not experienced childhood trauma; 26,000 will attempt suicide; 20,800 may fall into alcoholism; and an alarming 40,700 will be victims of rape in adulthood. Moreover, a staggering 160,400 will suffer from mental health disorders, creating pathways to life-threatening metabolic illnesses such as heart disease, cancer, stroke, and diabetes.

Nowhere is there a greater example of the destruction and disintegration created by childhood trauma than in the lives of foster children.

The Revolving Door: When Foster Parents Give Up

Here is a statistic that should stop every policymaker in their tracks: **76% of placement disruptions are due to foster parents' inability or unwillingness to continue fostering.**[91]

Not the child's fault. Not a change in circumstances. Three out of four times a foster placement fails, it fails because the foster parents gave up.

And they give up in staggering numbers. Nationally, thirty to fifty percent of foster families quit fostering every single year.[92] More than half of all foster parents report wanting to quit at some point. The single most common reason foster parents request that a child be removed from their home? Aggressive behaviors—the very behaviors that are predictable, understandable responses to the trauma these children have experienced.[93]

Think about what this means for a child like Darius. He enters the system already carrying wounds from abuse and neglect. His brain has been rewired for survival. He displays behaviors that confuse and frighten adults who don't understand what they're seeing. And so he is moved. Again and again and again.

Each Move Is a New Wound

Each move is a new trauma. Each time a foster family "gives him back," it confirms what his wounded brain already believes: He is unlovable, he is too much, he will always be abandoned. The research is unambiguous: Children who experience four or more placement moves are over ninety percent likely to end up in the juvenile justice system.[94] We are not just failing to help these children—we are actively making them worse.

But here is what the research also shows: *Quality training and support for foster parents can prevent placement disruption.*[91] When foster parents understand trauma neurobiology—when they know why a child hoards food or flinches at sudden movements or rages when asked simple questions—they can respond therapeutically rather than taking it personally. When they have co-regulation skills, they can help a dysregulated child return to calm rather than escalating the situation. When they are surrounded by a support network that provides respite and encouragement, they can endure the hard days without burning out.

Currently, only thirty-three percent of foster parents feel they received adequate training for the emotional challenges of fostering.[93] We are sending unprepared people into one of the hardest jobs imaginable—and then blaming them when they fail. The solution is not to recruit more foster parents to replace the ones who quit. The solution is to equip foster parents to succeed *before* their first placement, so they don't quit, so placements don't disrupt, so children stop accumulating new traumas in the very system designed to protect them.

What the ACE Score Doesn't Tell You

As we explored earlier in this book, the Adverse Childhood Experiences assessment counts *types* of trauma—neglect, physical abuse, sexual abuse, household dysfunction, and so on. A person can score anywhere from zero to ten, with higher scores indicating exposure to more categories of adversity.[8]

But here is what the ACE score fails to capture: **intensity, frequency, and duration.**

Consider two children, both with an ACE score of one for neglect. The first child had an inattentive, mildly depressive mother who sometimes forgot to pack lunch. The second child was removed from a home of severe neglect, placed in foster care, bounced through eight different placements over six years, and experienced the repeated trauma of adults promising to love them and then giving them away.

Same ACE score. Vastly different trauma load.

This is why foster children represent the most severely traumatized population we have. It's not just that they experienced adverse childhood experiences before entering care—it's that *the care system itself often compounds their trauma.* Every placement disruption is a new abandonment. Every new home is a new environment where they must assess threats, learn new rules, grieve what they've lost. The cumulative weight of this—what researchers call *allostatic load*—becomes almost unbearable.[95]

Allostatic load is the biological term for the wear and tear on the body from chronic, repeated stress. It shows up in elevated cortisol, inflammation, compromised immune function, cardiovascular strain.[94] A child with eight foster placements doesn't just have psychological wounds—their body has been under siege for years. Their nervous system has been in survival mode so long it has forgotten how to rest.

Research shows that children entering foster care have average ACE scores of five or higher.[8] Their brains have been neurobiologically altered by chronic stress. As we discussed in earlier chapters, the hippocampus is compromised. The prefrontal cortex is underdeveloped. The amygdala is hyperactive. Their nervous systems are locked in fight-or-flight.[96]

These are not "bad kids" with "behavioral problems." These are wounded children whose brains have adapted to survive environments of chaos and danger. The child who hoards food remembers starvation. The child who lies reflexively learned that truth-telling got them hurt. The teenager who rages is experiencing nervous system dysregulation, not defiance.[17]

This is the population we are handing to foster parents with a brief orientation and a prayer. This is why love alone is not enough. These children carry trauma loads that would break most adults—and we expect untrained caregivers to somehow absorb and heal that pain through good intentions. It is a setup for failure. And when the placement inevitably disrupts, the child's allostatic load increases again, the biological damage deepens, and the cycle continues.

The Pipeline: From Foster Care to Prison

The connection between trauma and systemic failures in the foster care system creates significant barriers to successful adulthood for these young people. The foster care-to-prison pipeline serves as a stark illustration of how these early adversities can funnel children into the criminal legal system, with research indicating that over eighty percent of foster youth will interact with law enforcement by the time they reach age eighteen.[90]

These experiences leave foster children grappling with stigmas and reinforce the belief that they are "trouble-makers" or "lost causes," deepening their sense of abandonment, hopelessness, and worthlessness. Without intervention and healing, these children will become adults who have a strong possibility of perpetuating generational trauma on their own children.

Every child who ages out of foster care into homelessness or addiction or prison represents a preventable tragedy. Every foster placement that fails because the parents weren't trained is a wound we inflicted. Every dollar spent on downstream crisis intervention is a dollar that could have been invested in upstream prevention.

We've Been Treating Symptoms, Not the Cause

For decades, we have approached foster care as a logistics problem. Not enough foster homes. Not enough social workers. Not enough funding. So we recruited more families, hired more caseworkers, allocated more dollars.

We were wrong. Foster care is not fundamentally a logistics problem. **It is a trauma problem.** And until we treat it as such, no amount of funding or infrastructure will change the outcomes.

We have spent billions of dollars on this crisis. We have built infrastructure. We have launched initiatives. We have held conferences and formed committees and published reports. And yet the outcomes remain catastrophic. Why? Because we have been treating symptoms while the disease rages unchecked.

The Solution We've Been Missing: Becoming Trauma-Responsive

The solution is not more of the same. The solution is fundamentally different: we must become **trauma-responsive.**

Not trauma-informed—a term that has been diluted to meaninglessness through overuse. Being "trauma-informed" means attending a workshop and putting a poster on the wall. It means awareness without action, knowledge without transformation.

Being trauma-responsive means fundamentally changing how we operate. It means training foster parents not just to love traumatized children, but to understand the neurobiology driving their behaviors and respond therapeutically rather than punitively. It means teaching social workers to recognize trauma responses and avoid re-traumatization. It means equipping teachers, judges, court staff—everyone who touches a child in crisis—with the skills to help rather than harm.

Trauma-informed is knowing. Trauma-responsive is doing. We have plenty of the former. We desperately need the latter.

The Power of the States

Here is something most people don't realize about the foster care system: it is not a federal system. It is a state system. Every state in America has direct jurisdiction over the agencies and professions that touch a foster child's life. The state controls licensing for social workers. The state controls licensing for teachers. The state controls the family court system and the judges who preside over custody decisions. And in most states, the state controls the requirements for becoming a licensed foster parent.

This means that a single governor, with the support of the state legislature, has the authority to fundamentally transform how every professional in the child welfare ecosystem is trained. A single legislative act could mandate trauma-responsive certification for every social worker, every teacher, every juvenile court judge, and every foster parent in the state. No federal legislation required. No partisan gridlock. No waiting for Washington.

The states that move first will become models for the nation. They will demonstrate that becoming trauma-responsive is not only morally imperative but practically achievable—and the results will speak for themselves in reduced placement disruptions, reduced incarceration, reduced homelessness, and most importantly, in children who are finally given the chance to heal.

Many states already have the infrastructure in place. They have faith-based networks, community organizations, and governmental structures that are ready to be leveraged. They have the funding committed to foster care reform. What has been missing is a comprehensive strategy to address the biological reality of childhood trauma. That strategy now exists.

A Three-Part Strategy

First, we must train and certify foster parents before their first placement. Not a two-hour orientation. Real training in trauma neurobiology, nervous system regulation, co-regulation techniques, and therapeutic responses to trauma behaviors. We don't let people practice medicine or law or teach in classrooms without certification.

Why do we hand traumatized children to adults with nothing but good intentions?

Second, we must certify the professionals. Every social worker, every teacher, every juvenile court judge and court staff member who interacts with children in crisis should be required to complete trauma-responsive certification. The states control licensing for all these professions. A single legislative act could mandate this training across the entire child welfare ecosystem.

Third, we must mobilize the churches. Faith communities have something government can never provide: relationship. Belonging. Extended family. If we can train churches to be trauma-responsive—to recognize trauma, to avoid re-traumatization, to support foster families and at-risk parents—we unlock an army of healers that no government program can replicate.

Why Churches Are Essential

I am not a pastor. I am an engineer, an inventor, a businessman. But I have come to believe that the church may be the single most important institution in solving the foster care crisis—if it is equipped to respond to trauma.

Many trauma survivors turn to faith communities seeking healing. The church offers what they desperately need: unconditional love, community, meaning, hope. But too often, well-meaning pastors and ministry leaders, untrained in trauma's neurobiological effects, inadvertently cause harm. They tell survivors to "pray harder" or "forgive and move on" without understanding that trauma creates wounds that don't respond to spiritual disciplines alone. They interpret trauma behaviors as spiritual failures rather than survival adaptations.

The church doesn't need to become a therapy clinic. But it does need to become trauma-responsive—able to recognize trauma, avoid re-traumatization, and connect survivors with appropriate resources while providing the relational support that only faith communities can offer.

Imagine if every church that hosts a foster care ministry first certified its ministers, counselors, and volunteers in trauma-responsive care. Imagine if every faith-based foster family received real training before their first placement. Imagine if churches became not just recruiters of foster parents, but *trainers and supporters* of foster parents—surrounding them with community, respite, and ongoing education.

The Stakes Could Not Be Higher

As I've documented throughout this book, childhood trauma accounts for approximately 1,401 American deaths every day. Not from the trauma itself—from its downstream effects: heart disease, addiction, suicide, stroke, diabetes, and more. Childhood trauma is not merely correlated with these leading causes of death. It is the root cause.

Foster children carry some of the highest trauma loads of any population. They enter the system already wounded. And then, too often, the system wounds them further—through placement disruptions, through professionals who don't understand trauma, through foster parents who burn out because they were never equipped to succeed.

Addressing the multitude of unique issues faced by foster children requires systemic change within the foster care system itself. Emphasis must be placed on providing trauma-responsive care and adequate resources for foster families, which includes training programs that help caregivers understand the emotional and psychological needs of the children in their care. Additionally, implementing supportive measures—such as educational opportunities, mental health services, and job training programs—can mitigate some damaging effects of their early experiences, thus breaking the cycle of adversity.

Darius Deserved Better

I lost two brothers to heroin addiction. Adam and Patrick died because their childhood trauma went unrecognized and untreated for decades. I didn't understand what had happened to them—what had happened to all of us—until I was seventy-two years old, writing a memoir about growing up as one of fourteen children in Kankakee, Illinois.

What I discovered changed everything. The "tough childhood" we thought we'd survived was actually complex trauma. The addiction, the broken relationships, the health problems that plagued my family—all of it traced back to adverse childhood experiences that no one had a name for, much less a solution to.

I can't go back and save my brothers. But I can fight to ensure that the next generation of traumatized children—including the more than 400,000 currently in America's foster care system—gets something we never had: adults who understand what happened to them and know how to help them heal.

Darius deserved better. So do the thousands of children who will enter foster care this year. So do the foster parents who will try and fail because no one taught them what they needed to know.

The solution is not to build more foster homes—but to equip the foster parents in those homes to actually heal wounded children. Not to hire more social workers—but to train those social workers to recognize and respond to trauma. Not to spend more money—but to spend it on root causes instead of symptoms. And just maybe, in a small but powerful way, we begin to disrupt generational trauma.

Book II
The Path Behind & the Road Ahead

In Book II, we examine how humanity has reached a point where childhood trauma impacts over two-thirds of the population. We'll examine the societal, cultural, and historical shifts that have contributed to this staggering prevalence.

The journey takes us through multiple perspectives—from anthropological insights into how societies have evolved in their treatment of children, to psychological understanding of how trauma patterns become embedded in communities. We'll investigate how modern pressures, changing family structures, and technological advances have potentially contributed to this crisis.

Beyond understanding the "how," we'll conduct a thorough examination of current healing approaches—celebrating what works while honestly confronting what doesn't. Drawing from cutting-edge research and real-world applications, we'll explore why certain interventions succeed while others fall short, providing insights for both professionals and survivors.

Perhaps most intriguingly, we'll delve into what I call the "resilience paradox"—the phenomenon where some individuals emerge from trauma with remarkable strength while others struggle to cope. Through compelling case studies and scientific research, we'll unravel the inter-action of factors that influence these divergent outcomes, from genetic predisposition to environmental support systems.

This section serves not just as historical analysis but as a foundation for understanding how we can better address childhood trauma moving forward. I believe that when we understand where we've been and what we've learned, we can more effectively chart the course toward healing and prevention.

CHAPTER EIGHTEEN

How Did We Get Here?

"There can be no keener revelation of a society's soul than
the way it treats its children."

—Nelson Mandela

OVER THE PAST TWO years I found myself immersed in research that illuminated the stark realities of childhood trauma. Among the more than 30 books I consumed, one stood out as profoundly transformative: *The Adverse Childhood Experiences Recovery Workbook* by Glenn R. Schiraldi, PhD. His insights on trauma recovery and resilience resonated deeply, reshaping my understanding of the pervasive nature of this crisis.

In the wake of my research, I was left with three urgent questions I felt compelled to pose to Dr. Schiraldi:

1. Is the problem as widespread and dire as your writings suggest? If so,
2. How did humanity arrive at a point where the pervasive experiences of neglect, abuse, and dysfunctional families have become so commonplace for our children?

3. What accounts for the differing paths of my siblings and me in coping with the weight of childhood trauma—why did some of us thrive, while others collapsed?

With a blend of trepidation and hope, I reached out to Dr. Schiraldi via email, sharing my journey and aspirations for my book. My previous attempts to connect with authors and experts had often been met with silence, so I tempered my expectations. To my astonishment, within minutes, my phone rang; it was an enthusiastic call from Dr. Schiraldi himself. He not only expressed appreciation for my work and my inquiries but also graciously agreed to read my manuscript and provide feedback. I am honored to feature his words on the cover of *The Kite That Couldn't Fly*, a testament to our budding friendship. Recently, Dr. Schiraldi offered me a momentous compliment, introducing me to someone as his colleague.

As I set my sights on writing *Greater Than Gravity*, I had the privilege of interviewing Dr. Schiraldi again, this time in person, where I was able to revisit those pivotal questions, alongside a host of others that had emerged through my research. The very next day, I finalized the outline for *Greater Than Gravity* and began writing.

What follows in this chapter is heavily informed by that enlightening interview, supplemented by insights from a wide spectrum of experts, including anthropologists, sociologists, theologians, and thought leaders. Together, we strive to answer the urgent question:

"How has civilization evolved to inflict such profound devastation on our children?"

It is important to note that there are no absolute answers here. I am simply gathering and synthesizing diverse perspectives. This discussion is organized by discipline—anthropology, sociology, and theology—culminating in my personal reflections. The answers to this question range from a simple one or two sentences to an extremely complex, multi-faceted answer, which I believe is required to attempt to answer the question.

Anthropological Perspective

Anthropologists often concentrate on the evolutionary, historical, and cultural dimensions of human societies. They typically explore how cultures develop over time, examining rituals, customs, and social structures through ethnographic methods. Their work may span time and societies, looking at the broader human experience and how past events shape present realities.

I posed the question, "How would you explain how civilization evolved to a place where 70% of all adults are suffering from some form of childhood trauma?" In my extensive research to understand how civilization evolved to a place where 70% of adults suffer from childhood trauma, I consulted numerous anthropological studies and academic works.

My research revealed that childhood trauma isn't just a modern phenomenon but has deep historical roots across various civilizations where societal structures often placed children in vulnerable positions. I discovered compelling evidence about cultural transmission—how traumatic patterns get passed down through generations, shaping parenting styles and community support systems.

The academic literature I studied highlighted how social hierarchies and systemic inequalities create environments where stressors are magnified for children. From an evolutionary standpoint, the research explains how our biological stress responses, which once helped us survive, can be overwhelmed by modern traumas.

Finally, my investigation uncovered how globalization and modernization have disrupted traditional support systems that previously protected children, potentially explaining the high prevalence of childhood trauma we see today.

What emerged was a nuanced understanding that draws from evolutionary history, social structures, and cultural contexts.

Historical Context: The anthropologists emphasized that childhood trauma is not a modern phenomenon but has deep roots in human history. They noted that throughout various periods and civilizations, societal structures often placed children in vulnerable positions, whether through warfare, economic hardship, or unstable family dynamics. These historical contexts laid the groundwork for patterns of behavior and societal norms that persist today.[97]

Cultural Transmission: A key point raised was the concept of cultural transmission—the idea that behaviors, beliefs, and norms are passed down through generations. They highlighted that trauma experienced by previous generations can shape parenting styles, societal expectations, and community support systems. The absence of nurturing environments or the normalization of violence and neglect can perpetuate cycles of trauma, leaving subsequent generations to grapple with its consequences.[98]

Social Hierarchies & Inequities: The anthropologists discussed how social hierarchies and systemic inequalities contribute to the prevalence of childhood trauma. Factors such as poverty, marginalization, and discrimination create environments where stressors are magnified, leading to emotional, physical, and psychological harm in children. They posited that these inequities have persisted across cultures and time, creating a context in which trauma proliferates.[99]

Evolutionary Perspectives: From an evolutionary standpoint, the anthropologists explored the impact of biological and neurological responses to stress. They explained that early human environments often required resilience to survive adversity. However, in modern contexts, heightened exposure to trauma can overwhelm these adaptive responses, resulting in lasting psychological effects. This evolutionary lens suggests that while humans are designed to cope with challenges, the complexities of contemporary life may exceed our inherent capacities for resilience.[100]

Globalization & Modernization: Finally, the group addressed the impact of globalization and modernization on childhood experiences. They indicated that rapid changes in societal structures, family dynamics, and community cohesion can disrupt traditional support systems that previously buffered children from trauma. This dislocation may lead to increased rates of neglect, abuse, and emotional disconnection, further exacerbating the prevalence of childhood trauma across diverse populations.[101]

It was like these experts had prepared their whole life to answer this one question. Interestingly, none of them were surprised by my findings on the prevalence of childhood trauma.

While both anthropologists and sociologists study human behavior and societies, their approaches and areas of focus diverge significantly.

Sociological Perspective

Sociologists focus more on social behavior within contemporary societies, analyzing structures, institutions, and relationships. They often use statistical methods, surveys, and observational studies to understand social phenomena like class, race, gender, and the dynamics of group behavior. Sociology tends to emphasize current social systems and the interactions within them, aiming to understand how they contribute to social problems, including violence, inequality, and trauma.

Using the same hypothetical question, "How would you explain how civilization evolved to a place where 70% of all adults are suffering from some form of childhood trauma?" here is a summary of what I discovered from a sociological perspective:

Institutionalized Inequality: The sociologists pointed to the structural inequalities embedded within social institutions—such as family, education, and healthcare—that have historically marginalized certain groups. They argued that systemic barriers based on socio-economic status, race, and gender create environments where childhood trauma is likely to occur, as disadvantaged communities often lack resources and support systems to shield children from harm.[102]

Socialization & Norms: The group emphasized the role of socialization in shaping attitudes towards childhood and parenting. They noted that prevailing cultural norms often dictate acceptable forms of discipline and parenting styles. In environments where aggression or neglect is normalized, children are more likely to experience trauma. The sociologists highlighted the need to reframe these norms toward fostering nurturing and supportive environments for all children.[103]

Impact of Social Change: The group of sociologists also highlighted how rapid social changes, such as urbanization, globalization, and technological advancement, disrupt traditional family structures and community cohesion. They suggested that as families become more isolated, the social support systems that historically helped protect children from trauma weaken. These shifts can lead to increased stress and disconnection, making children more vulnerable to adverse experiences.[104]

Media & Exposure to Violence: The role of media and technology was another focal point of discussion. The sociologists noted that the pervasive exposure to violence and trauma through various forms of media can desensitize individuals and contribute to a cycle of aggression and neglect. This exposure can diminish empathy and normalize harmful behaviors in both children and adults, perpetuating a culture where trauma proliferates.[105]

Intergenerational Transmission of Trauma: Finally, the panel addressed the concept of intergenerational trauma, explaining how the effects of childhood trauma can ripple through families and communities. They discussed how unresolved trauma can affect parenting styles, leading to a continuation of adverse experiences. This cyclical nature emphasizes the importance of addressing trauma at every level of society to break the cycle and promote healing.[106]

In my interview with Dr. Cecilia Garza, a sociologist at the Laredo Diploma Foundation, her response to my question about the prevalence of childhood trauma was as immediate as it was unsettling.

"It's our evolution to materialism," she declared, her eyes reflecting the gravity of her conviction. "We've transformed from a society that prioritized nurturing children to one obsessed with acquisition."

She leaned forward, her voice dropping to emphasize each word. "Parents today aren't just working to provide necessities—they're chasing an endless cycle of consumption. The constant pursuit of more—more house, more car, more status—has created a vacuum where childhood development should be."

Dr. Garza explained that this shift represents more than just changing values; it's a fundamental restructuring of our social architecture. The time, energy, and emotional presence that children require has been systematically redirected toward material gain—a trade-off with consequences we're only beginning to fully comprehend.

"When we choose acquisition over attention," she concluded, "we're essentially telling our children that things matter more than their development. And that message—that profound displacement of priorities—lies at the heart of our trauma epidemic."

Sociologists provide a comprehensive analysis of how social structures, norms, and changes contribute to the widespread prevalence of childhood trauma. I expected simpler answers—hoping for one area we could use a huge lever on to enact change and prevention. Instead, the problem and the answers grew in complexity.

Their insights call for a critical examination of the existing social systems and advocate for a collective effort to cultivate environments that prioritize the well-being of all children, inviting a transformation in societal attitudes toward childhood and trauma recovery.

Let's move from an evolutionary lens to the spiritual.

Theological Perspectives

I am a Christian and have followed the teachings of Jesus Christ my entire life.

When examining the issue of childhood trauma through a theological lens, we must engage with the concepts of morality, ethics, and the spiritual understanding of human suffering. Different religious perspectives address the questions of right and wrong, good and bad, as they seek to explain the presence of evil, suffering, and injustice in the world. In this context, theologians aim to understand how spiritual beliefs, practices, and narratives shape our responses to trauma and inform our responsibilities towards the vulnerable, especially children.

Each tradition offers unique insights into human suffering and the paths toward healing, redemption, and moral responsibility.

Here's how various theological perspectives from major religions—including Christianity, Judaism, Islam, Hinduism, and Buddhism—responded to the question, "How would you explain how civilization evolved to a place where 70% of all adults are suffering from some form of childhood trauma?"

Christianity

Christian theologians frame the prevalence of childhood trauma within a complex theological landscape that begins with the doctrine of original sin and humanity's fallen nature. For centuries, Christian thought has wrestled with the profound question of why innocent children suffer in a world created by a loving God.

At its foundation, Christian theology points to the fracturing of God's perfect creation through humanity's disobedience. The Garden of Eden narrative represents not just a historical event but an archetypal break in the divine ordering of relationships—between humans and God, between people, and within the human heart itself. This primordial rupture, theologians argue, continues to reverberate through generations, manifesting in the broken systems and relationships that often give rise to childhood trauma.

Renowned theologian Reinhold Niebuhr described sin as "the pride which confuses our finitude with the ultimate and makes our partial perspective an absolute one." This prideful distortion leads to what many Christian thinkers identify as the root causes of childhood trauma: the pursuit of power over others, moral abdication of responsibility toward the vulnerable, and the elevation of self-interest above the protection of children.

The Catholic tradition, while acknowledging the role of human sinfulness, also emphasizes what Pope Francis calls "structural sins"—institutionalized patterns of injustice that enable child suffering. These include economic systems that prioritize profit over family well-being, social structures that isolate parents from support networks, and cultural values that diminish the sacred worth of childhood.

Protestant perspectives often highlight the personal moral failure of caregivers, pointing to scriptural imperatives like Jesus's stern warning that "whoever causes one of these little ones to stumble, it would be better for them if a millstone were hung around their neck and they were thrown into the sea." This represents both the gravity of harm to children and God's special concern for their protection.

Orthodox Christian thought adds the dimension of spiritual warfare, suggesting that forces of darkness specifically target the innocent to perpetuate cycles of suffering and alienation from God. In this view, childhood trauma reflects not just human failing but a cosmic battle in which children become casualties.

Yet across these perspectives runs a thread of hope distinctive to Christian theology: the belief in redemption and restoration. The central Christian narrative of a God who enters into human suffering through the incarnation offers a counterpoint to despair. The cross becomes a symbol that God does not stand aloof from trauma but bears it, transforms it, and ultimately promises healing through the power of resurrection.

As theologian Jürgen Moltmann writes, "God weeps with us so that we may someday laugh with him." This framing suggests that while sin and moral failure indeed contribute fundamentally to childhood trauma, they do not have the final word in the Christian understanding of human suffering or divine purpose.

Judaism

Jewish theologians approach the topic by emphasizing the concept of *Tikkun Olam*, or "repairing the world," which compels individuals and communities to take action against suffering. They recognize that childhood trauma often stems from systemic injustices, and therefore, community responsibility is crucial. The Jewish faith underscores the importance of relationships and covenantal obligations—parents, communities, and society at large have the responsibility to nurture and protect children. Through teachings of compassion and justice found in the Torah and Talmud, Jews emphasize the need for social action and support systems to prevent trauma and promote healing.

Islam

In Islam, theologians explain the prevalence of childhood trauma through the lens of *fitrah*, or the inherent nature of humans created by Allah. They argue that while humans are born pure, societal and familial dysfunction can lead to trauma. Islamic teachings emphasize mercy, compassion, and the responsibility of individuals towards their families and communities. Scholars often reference the *Hadiths* of the Prophet Muhammad, which stress kindness towards children, reminding that those who cause harm to the innocent will face severe consequences. There is a strong call within Islam to address injustices and work towards community welfare, with faith as a source of resilience and hope.

Hinduism

Hindu theologians view childhood trauma in the context of karma and the cycle of *samsara* (rebirth). They explain that the experiences of trauma could be a product of accumulated karmic influences from past lives or the current life. However, this perspective must be balanced with the belief in the responsibilities of parents and society in creating nurturing environments for children. Hinduism teaches the importance of *dharma*, or duty, prompting families and communities to uphold their responsibilities to prevent harm to children and support healing through practices like prayer, meditation, and community service.

Buddhism

Buddhist theologians focus on the nature of suffering as articulated in the Four Noble Truths. They explain that *dukkha* (suffering) is an inherent part of life but can be alleviated through compassion, mindfulness, and understanding. The interconnectedness of all beings means that trauma experienced by children affects everyone. Buddhists emphasize the importance of *metta* (loving-kindness) and *karuna* (compassion) as responses to trauma, advocating for nurturing environments for vulnerable populations. They also encourage healing through mindfulness practices, teachings on impermanence, and compassionate action.

All religions believe causing and perpetuating childhood trauma is wrong, and many experts believe spirituality is a critical component required for healing from childhood trauma. Ironically, I believe churches are full of those both committing and suffering from childhood trauma. That being said, I still appreciate the diverse insights of different theological perspectives on good and evil, moral responsibility, and the nature of human suffering.

Each perspective emphasizes community support, compassion, and the moral imperative to protect and nurture children, often with strong warnings against harming the innocent. The teachings of Christ remind believers of their solemn obligation to protect children and act justly. All religious groups could more strongly advocate for a commitment to upholding the sanctity of childhood by actively working to reduce trauma and create environments that foster healing, hope, and resilience that promote the well-being of future generations.

My Answer

How do I explain the prevalence of childhood trauma and its devastating effects? Why do I believe we've evolved into a society where 70% of us experience this toxic trauma? I have strong opinions on the matter, but I recognize that I am biased, and my perspective represents just one view among many.

From a Christian perspective, faith in Christ and His teachings inherently includes belief in the existence of Satan and his insidious desire to destroy lives. What more devious method could there be to undermine humanity than the implantation of the poisonous seed of childhood trauma?

A powerful scripture that resonates with the darker forces at play in our world is found in 1 Peter 5:8: *"Be alert and of sober mind. Your enemy the devil prowls around like a roaring lion looking for someone to devour."* This vivid imagery highlights a metaphor for the very real threat posed by the cycle of trauma we see around us and underscores the urgent need for awareness, compassion, and action.

Generational Trauma

In my opinion, one of the most distressing aspects of this cycle is generational trauma, which I often describe as "the gift that keeps taking." Research indicates about 40% of those who experience childhood trauma go on to neglect or abuse their own children. Considering there are an estimated 180 million adults in the US alone who have experienced childhood trauma, that means around 72 million adults may unwittingly continue this cycle. If we assume each of these adults has on average two children, we find a grim projection: Approximately 144 million children may also suffer from childhood trauma.

Childhood trauma isn't just a recent problem—it's deeply rooted in the very fabric of human history, woven through generations and civilizations across thousands of years. This stubborn pattern has been strengthened through cultural transmission, reinforced by social inequalities, and accelerated by modern disruptions to traditional family structures. The fact that 70% of adults today carry childhood wounds reveals the enormous mountain we must climb. We're not just addressing individual healing but confronting ancient patterns embedded in how we parent, structure our communities, and treat our most vulnerable. This isn't a simple fix—it's about reimagining human relationships that have developed over millennia. The depth and persistence of childhood trauma throughout human history shows us we're tackling one of humanity's most enduring and complex challenges.

As John Steinbeck eloquently framed it in *East of Eden*, we are all born into a world of tests and trials, and our goal is to climb over the fence that separates us from the bad. This struggle is not just a personal one; it reflects the larger societal battle between nurturing environments and those that perpetuate harm.

CHAPTER NINETEEN

What's Not Working

"Every misstep is a steppingstone; understanding what doesn't work illuminates the path to what will."

–Michael Menard

GIVEN THE TRAVESTIES AND the size of what I now hope you see as the crisis, there is obviously so much that is not working to address the destruction and disintegration. As we continue with the critical topic of childhood trauma, it is essential to recognize that our society, sadly and surprisingly, is still in the budding stages of understanding and addressing this epidemic.

To illustrate our current state, we can draw a parallel to the fight against infectious diseases around the 1900's. In our efforts to combat childhood trauma, we might liken our progress to being at the very first phase: the hand-washing stage. Just as effective hand hygiene was once simply a foundational practice in preventing illness, raising awareness and initiating conversations around childhood trauma is a necessary, albeit insufficient, starting point.

Despite the strides made in the fields of mental health, education, and social services, we have yet to implement comprehensive and effective strategies that can genuinely disrupt the cycle of childhood trauma. As a society, we lack a shared understanding of childhood trauma and the pervasive nature of its associated problems. The enormity of the challenge we face signals a pressing need for more robust interventions, proactive prevention measures, and systemic changes in how we approach and understand childhood trauma.

I have an admittedly simplistic view on the three areas of effort required to end childhood trauma: Awareness, Healing Interventions, and Prevention.

First, we will explore a short list of what I believe isn't working with our current efforts to address childhood trauma. This examination will shed light on the gaps in knowledge, policy, and practice that undermine our ability to protect vulnerable children and heal those who have already suffered. In doing so, I hope to foster a clearer vision of the steps necessary to move beyond mere acknowledgment and begin the transformative work required to create a safer, healthier future for children and all sufferers of childhood trauma—one that addresses not only the symptoms of trauma but also its root causes.

Only by recognizing what is failing can we begin to innovate new approaches and cultivate effective solutions that can truly heal the wounds of childhood trauma and reduce its far-reaching impact on individuals and humanity.

Before we continue, I must acknowledge there *are* people and organizations that are performing groundbreaking, beautiful work. They are doing things that are working, things we need to learn from and leverage. Those guiding lights will be highlighted in the following chapter.

Awareness

Awareness is the crucial first step in driving any meaningful change, yet when it comes to the issue of childhood trauma, we find ourselves gravely lacking. Despite ongoing efforts to shed light on various societal issues, the conversation surrounding childhood trauma remains disproportionately muted. It's often overshadowed by more visible crises—poverty, war, racism, and other pressing global challenges. However, the reality is that the ramifications of childhood trauma ripple through society, affecting not only the individuals who endure it but also the broader community and future generations.

Until I wrote my memoir at the age of 72, I had no idea that what my siblings and I had experienced throughout our childhoods was classified as complex childhood trauma. I navigated life believing that our struggles were isolated events or personal failings, only to learn later that they aligned with a broader, alarming pattern of experiences that millions—even billions—endure. This revelation was not just enlightening; it was essential for my healing. It speaks volumes about the gaps in awareness that exist even among those who have lived through traumatic experiences. If individuals like me, who have faced childhood trauma, can go so long without recognizing it as such, how can we expect society at large to understand its magnitude?

In my search for lists outlining the top issues facing humanity, I discovered that poverty, war, obesity, drug abuse, and racism dominate these discussions, while the profound impact of childhood trauma remains conspicuously absent. Despite research showing that the prevalence of childhood trauma—and its long-term effects—exceeds that of cancer, heart disease, diabetes, and stroke combined, it fails to secure a place in the national or global discourse. How can this be? This oversight is not merely a missed opportunity; it is a glaring indication of the systemic neglect of childhood trauma.

The evidence is clear: Increased awareness could lead to transformative changes in how we address not only individual mental health struggles but also societal well-being. Yet, there is an obvious lack of understanding and recognition of childhood trauma in both public and private sectors. Health care providers often overlook the signs of trauma in their patients, educators may remain uninformed about the profound effects of adverse childhood experiences on learning and behavior, and communities as a whole often do not realize the deep-seated roots of dysfunction and violence that can stem from unresolved childhood trauma.

The emotional and psychological toll of childhood trauma is frequently dismissed or rationalized, leading to stigmatization rather than empathy. This lack of awareness creates barriers to advocacy and impedes the development of effective interventions. Siloed discussions about trauma further isolate survivors, perpetuating the myth that trauma is a personal struggle rather than a communal concern that demands collective action.

The arena of awareness surrounding childhood trauma is rife with shortcomings. While some efforts are underway to raise consciousness about this widespread issue, the prevailing narrative remains grossly insufficient. Without a concerted focus on elevating awareness, we risk allowing a critical aspect of human suffering to remain in the shadows, hidden and unaddressed. Until we are willing to acknowledge childhood trauma as a fundamental issue affecting lives and entire societies, meaningful changes in healing interventions and preventative measures will remain just out of reach.

How can we change something we are not even aware of?

Healing Interventions

In Book I, we explored the profound impact of toxic trauma on a child's mind and body, revealing the mental, physical, and social disintegration that can unexpectedly surface as these children move into adulthood. This upheaval occurs largely because the trauma and the resulting stress responses remain unresolved. While awareness of childhood trauma is an essential starting point, helping many individuals comprehend their experiences, it often falls short of providing the healing necessary to truly move forward.

For countless sufferers and survivors, understanding the effects of trauma is not enough; they require targeted healing interventions to address the complex disorders and illnesses that emerge because of their childhood experiences. In this chapter, I focus specifically on the mental health aspects of healing, examining the various therapeutic approaches designed to mitigate the psychological scars left by trauma, rather than delving into the physical or metabolic diseases that may also arise.

By zeroing in on the mental health dimension, we can better understand what is not working in our current healing practices and therapies. It is imperative that we critically assess the limitations of existing interventions, the gaps in accessibility and effectiveness, and the ways in which our societal understanding of trauma may obstruct pathways to genuine recovery. Only by identifying these shortcomings can we hope to develop more effective methods of healing that truly honor and support those affected by childhood trauma.

Healing from childhood trauma has proven to be a convoluted and often disappointing journey. With an estimated 21 million adults in the US experiencing at least one depressive episode in 2020, the link between childhood trauma and mental health conditions, particularly depression, is undeniable. The Adverse Childhood Experiences (ACEs) study found that 40% of depression cases in the US, translating to over 8 million adults, are attributed to childhood trauma.[8] Yet, despite the high prevalence of treatment, the effectiveness of these interventions raises serious questions about why healing is, for the most part, elusive.

The statistics are sobering: a study by the National Institute of Mental Health reports that two-thirds of individuals suffering from depression seek treatment, yet a longitudinal study spanning over a decade revealed that 90% of participants reported ongoing symptoms, fluctuating between episodes of major depression and enduring low-grade afflictio ns.[107] This study is not an outlier; it reflects a broader reality in mental health treatment. Most disturbed individuals do not simply experience even temporary relief but instead face a chronic, episodic struggle.

So, what happens to all these people who get treatment for depression? Do they get better—and most importantly, stay better—over the long run?

In an attempt to answer this question, researchers embarked on an extensive 12-year study, enlisting individuals seeking treatment from five esteemed academic medical centers. Twelve years of insight were gleaned from this investigation, which involved 431 participants whose symptoms were diligently assessed on a weekly basis.[107]

The results were striking—despite receiving treatment, a staggering 90% of these individuals reported persistent depressive symptoms after treatment. Over the course of the study, participants experienced symptoms of depression 59% of the time, illustrating a haunting fluctuation where relief would occasionally surface, only to be overshadowed by resurgent bouts of despair. In essence, the findings revealed a sobering reality: for the majority, depression was not simply a fleeting concern that could be cured. Instead, it manifested as a chronic yet episodic illness, characterized by low-grade, lingering discomfort or cyclical episodes of major depression.

Indeed, many turn to a plethora of therapeutic options—medications, psychotherapy, group therapy, meditation, and even invasive procedures like transcranial magnetic stimulation or electroconvulsive therapy. Despite these efforts, many find themselves labeled as having "treatment-resistant depression," while others may experience only transient relief that fails to translate into lasting recovery. The persistence of mental depression, alongside other mental illnesses, which remains the leading cause of disability worldwide, underscores the glaring inadequacy of current treatments.

Yet, the dissatisfaction with treatment does not stem solely from a lack of efficacy in medications or therapy techniques. In this layman's opinion, the root problem lies more profoundly in our approach to understanding and addressing mental disorders. Many patients, understandably frustrated, may blame themselves or misattribute their lack of progress to inadequacies in their treatment providers or diagnoses. In reality, the treatments often do not target the underlying causes of mental health issues; instead, they focus on symptom management. This symptomatic approach is particularly damaging when dealing with complex mental health issues associated with childhood trauma.

Understandably, some professionals in the mental health field may resist acknowledging these shortfalls for fear of instilling pessimism in patients. While the concern that such assessments might deter individuals from seeking help is valid, it also highlights the urgency to confront the limitations of current practices. Hiding these truths not only perpetuates a cycle of frustration for patients but perpetuates stigma. Patients who do not achieve improvement often internalize failure, doubting their resolve and commitment, while professionals grapple with the implications of treatment outcomes for their reputations. I've used the disorder of depression, but I believe the same issues are present across most all mental disorders and illnesses.

Dr. Tom Insel, the former director of the National Institute of Mental Health, has candidly stated that despite investment over $20 billion in understanding the neuroscience and genetics of mental disorders, the field has not significantly advanced outcomes for those suffering from mental illness or made any progress in reducing suicide and improving recovery rates.[108] One of the underlying failures is that systems frequently treat symptoms rather than the disorders themselves, neglecting the root causes of mental anguish that often stem from traumatic childhood experiences.

Where there is smoke…

I've heard Dr. Felitti use this analogy.

> "Imagine a fireman rushing to a blazing building, greeted
> not by flames, but by a thick cloud of smoke filling the air.
> Rather than addressing the core of the blaze—smothering
> the fire—he puts a fan on the smoke, desperately trying
> to clear the air. But in doing so, he only fans the flames
> to grow stronger and more destructive."

This is analogous to how many in the mental health community approach the effects of childhood trauma in adults. Rather than delving into the root causes—the buried flames of past pain and unresolved issues—they often treat the surface symptoms, like anxiety or depression and many times with drugs that further mask the root cause. But this approach doesn't extinguish the fire of trauma; it merely disperses the smoke, allowing the underlying distress to intensify.

To truly heal and prevent future devastation, we must be like that wise fireman who seeks the source of the fire, extinguishing it at the root, ensuring that the smoke doesn't return. In mental health, it's time we stop fanning the smoke and start putting out the fire.

In the landscape of mental health treatment, there appears to be a glaring disparity between the complexity of childhood trauma and the understanding held by many therapists and mental health practitioners. I believe that only a small percentage truly grasp the profound impact that early adverse experiences have on the brain and, more importantly, the nuanced interventions that can affect real change.

Too often, the prevailing approach to trauma is dominated by cognitive therapies—modalities that strive to alter thought patterns to influence emotions and behaviors. Many times this is called "Talk Therapy." While cognitive therapy can be beneficial for a variety of issues, it apparently falls short when confronting the deep-seated neurobiological effects of childhood trauma. Trauma impacts the brain at an elemental level, intertwining itself with our emotional regulation, attachment styles, and even our physiological responses to stress.

My brother Jamie is a great example. While suffering the symptoms of depression and anxiety over a long period, Jamie met with four different doctors and therapists seeking healing. Each time he was misdiagnosed with a different disorder and was treated with cognitive therapy and medication to treat the symptoms, which never made a difference, and at times made it all worse. It wasn't until Jamie stumbled upon the possibility that he was suffering from his childhood of complex trauma that he began a search for a therapist who specialized in childhood trauma recovery. Jamie found a therapist who treated him with EMDR therapy. After seven sessions, Jamie made transformational progress towards his healing journey.

Cognitive therapy may insufficiently address the embodied nature of trauma; it assumes that rational thought can easily override the visceral, often subconscious, reactions rooted in traumatic experiences. By focusing primarily on cognitive restructuring, practitioners may inadvertently ignore the need for deeper, somatic interventions that target the emotional and physiological remnants of trauma held within the body itself.

Trauma is not merely a matter of misaligned thoughts; it is an ingrained imprint on the brain and body that requires comprehensive, evidence-based approaches such as trauma-informed care and somatic therapies. Until a larger proportion of mental health professionals fully recognize and integrate these perspectives, many clients will continue to cycle through ineffective treatments, never truly healing from the remnants of their past, and worse yet may simply give up trying to find healing. In our pursuit of effective mental healthcare in general, we must strive to elevate the understanding and practice of trauma treatment, moving beyond surface-level remedies and toward strategies that recognize the full complexity of the human experience.

Prevention

The Adverse Childhood Experiences (ACEs) study, published in the late 1990s, revealed a stark truth about the prevalence of childhood trauma: over two-thirds of participants reported experiencing at least one adverse childhood event, and nearly one in five reported three or more. This landmark research illuminated the profound impact of childhood trauma on mental and physical health, underscoring its role as a precursor to a myriad of serious health issues, including depression, anxiety, substance abuse, chronic disease, and even premature death. Despite this pivotal understanding, one must ponder: What tangible progress has been made to prevent childhood trauma from perpetuating in our society? Regrettably, the answer remains unsettlingly clear: very little.

In the years following the ACEs study, there has been an increase in awareness surrounding the implications of childhood trauma. Initiatives have emerged, in disparate pockets, aimed at educating parents, caregivers, and professionals about the impacts of adverse experiences and the importance of trauma-informed care. However, these efforts have not translated into the necessary structural change or effective prevention strategies. We continue to witness alarming rates of abuse, neglect, and household dysfunction that inflict long-lasting damage on children. The systemic factors that contribute to childhood trauma, such as poverty, domestic violence, substance abuse, and social isolation, remain largely unaddressed.

I believe the primary barriers to meaningful progress is the fragmented nature of the services designed to support at-risk families. Mental health services, social work, and educational interventions often operate in silos, lacking the coordination necessary to provide comprehensive support to families grappling with adversity. This disconnect is compounded by grossly inadequate funding for social services, mental health resources, and preventive programs. Society's approach often reacts to trauma rather than addressing its root causes, leaving the most vulnerable populations to navigate an inadequate support system.

When I attempt to analyze public policy responses to the crisis, the picture becomes even bleaker. While there is lip service paid to the importance of protecting children, policies are inconsistently implemented and often fail to provide the robust support that families and communities need. A focus on punitive measures, such as child removal from homes, without addressing the underlying issues that lead to trauma—such as economic instability, lack of access to healthcare, and insufficient mental health resources—serves only to perpetuate the cycle of adversity.

In the realm of education, schools have begun to recognize the importance of addressing trauma; however, many still lack adequate training and resources to create truly trauma-informed environments. Teachers often find themselves overwhelmed with large class sizes and limited support, making it difficult to implement effective strategies for recognizing and responding to trauma in their students. Additionally, standardized testing and academic pressures do not account for the emotional and psychological toll trauma takes on a child's ability to learn.

Ultimately, all of us should be asking: Why have we failed to make significant strides in preventing childhood trauma despite the wealth of knowledge we possess about its prevalence and widespread destruction? The answer lies in a continued lack of prioritization on a societal level. We must confront the uncomfortable reality that childhood trauma is often viewed as a personal or family issue rather than a societal crisis. When the onus of addressing trauma is placed solely on the individual or family, without recognizing the broader systemic and cultural factors at play, we create an environment where prevention is not seen as a collective responsibility.

Are We Investing in Prevention?

Each year, US taxpayers allocate a staggering $5.4 billion to incarcerate individuals convicted of sex crimes against children. Currently, there are approximately 145,000 adults behind bars for these offenses, with most serving around eight years, and many, even longer. Over the course of this incarceration, we anticipate a total expenditure of about $49 billion on this group of sex offenders, with new inmates continuously entering the system. At first glance, this seems like a substantial investment in safeguarding children from abuse. However, by the time many of these offenders are processed by the criminal justice system, numerous children have already been harmed. Thus, a more significant consideration is the resources and effort we allocate toward prevention.

Up until recently, it is alarming to note that we dedicated almost no federal funding to the primary prevention of child sexual abuse. This oversight has led to a failure in supporting essential programs that could have intervened before the need for criminal justice involvement arose. Fortunately, there is a sliver of optimism on the horizon: Congress has started to shift its focus by including funding in the federal budget aimed specifically at preventing child sexual abuse. For instance, in 2023, a modest $2 million was earmarked for researching child sexual abuse prevention.

While this funding does represent a crucial step forward, it pales in comparison to our expenditures on punishment. For every dollar spent on prevention research, a staggering $2,700 goes toward incarceration. This figure merely scratches the surface, as it does not account for the significant costs associated with crime detection, prosecution, or the extensive post-release expenses related to parole, sex offender registration, and community notification. In simpler terms, we invest only 0.037% of what we spend on incarceration into prevention efforts. This disparity not only highlights the overwhelming focus on punitive responses but also emphasizes the urgent need to prioritize prevention initiatives to provide better protection for our children.

This disparity not only highlights the overwhelming focus on punitive responses but also emphasizes the urgent need to prioritize prevention initiatives to provide better protection for our children.

CHAPTER TWENTY

The Promise of Healing

"Hope is not pretending that troubles don't exist. It is the trust that they will not last forever, that hurts will be healed and difficulties overcome. It is faith that a source of strength and renewal lies within to lead us through the dark to the sunshine."

–Desmond Tutu

IN THIRD GRADE, WE are first introduced to the concept of negative numbers. The lesson typically begins with a simple scale—a horizontal line with zero at its center. To the left, negative values descend from -1 to -10, symbolizing increasingly severe states of hardship. To the right, positive values ascend from +1 to +10, representing degrees of well-being, joy, and fulfillment. Zero sits in the middle, epitomizing neutrality; it is neither negative nor positive.

Let us envision those grappling with childhood trauma as situated within this spectrum, often ensconced in the realm of negative numbers. The variety of experiences stemming from childhood trauma spans a vast range of disarray, where -10 symbolizes unimaginable despair, a place so dark that life itself feels unbearable. A -1, in contrast, might indicate a milder form of unease—a nagging discomfort, perhaps manifesting as mild depression or anxiety. On the scale, being to the left of zero signifies suffering and turmoil, while moving right, beyond zero signifies healing and hope.

For me, the promise of healing is an essential component of this discourse. I could not write *Greater Than Gravity* to merely shine a light on this challenging reality without also illuminating the path toward healing, that would have been irresponsible. Ideally, we might envision a world where every individual resides at +10, having discovered the keys to maximizing joy and fulfillment.

My intention is to guide those suffering toward at least reaching a state of neutrality—a solid zero on our numerical scale. Achieving neutrality means liberating yourself from the debilitating disorders and illnesses that result from childhood trauma. It is not about erasing painful memories, but instead about preventing them from casting a long shadow over your current life.

Reaching a neutral state does not automatically equate to happiness or a sense of purpose; those aspirations require a nuanced approach to a variety of personal factors. If this book can facilitate your journey from the painful, negative realm to a neutral position, we can celebrate a significant milestone together. However, in order to continue moving toward healing and happiness, you must practice consistent commitment and effort. This journey is not linear; it demands additional resources, knowledge, and determination.

Let me repeat myself here: I am neither a therapist nor do I possess any formal mental health or medical education. What you will find in this chapter and throughout this book is rooted in my personal journey, informed by research, and shaped by profound discussions with experts in the field of childhood trauma and recovery. Know that what is included here is limited to my knowledge and exposure and in no way should be viewed as the total list. It is not.

Navigating the path from trauma to healing is not just a possibility—it is a journey filled with promise that begins with awareness and leads to empowerment. As we explore what *is* working to foster healing from childhood trauma, remember that progress is always within reach, and the journey is worth taking.

The Foundation of Healing: Self-Care

Before we discuss interventions and recovery, let's first talk about doing all we can to prepare for and enable your journey to healing. Let's talk about what the experts like Drs. Schiraldi, Van der Kol, and Palmer have taught us about self-care. All three of these esteemed researchers and authors agree there are three aspects of life they believe have a strong correlation with healing from childhood trauma: sleep, nutrition, and exercise.

Dr. Schiraldi, in his book *The Adverse Childhood Experience Recovery Workbook*, sheds light on the profound impact that sleep has on emotional regulation and overall mental health. He emphasizes, "adequate sleep is essential for emotional and physical well-being; without it, our ability to process trauma diminishes."[9] Sleep is not merely a period of rest—it is a vital restorative process that allows our brains to consolidate memories and our bodies to heal. For survivors of childhood trauma, restorative sleep is crucial for managing anxiety, depression, and other mental health issues that often arise from past experiences. By prioritizing healthy sleep habits, individuals can enhance their resilience and cognitive functioning, thus enabling a more effective recovery process.

Nutrition, according to Dr. Palmer in *Brain Energy*, is another cornerstone of healing. He argues "what we consume significantly affects how our bodies function, including our mood and mental clarity."[20] A nutrient-rich diet provides the necessary building blocks for neurotransmitters and hormones that regulate mood and stress responses. Trauma can disrupt these systems, leading to imbalances that contribute to ongoing distress. Dr. Palmer advocates for whole foods, balanced meals, and hydration as the foundation of a healthy lifestyle, indicating that a well-nourished body can better cope with stressors and emotional challenges. This connection underscores the idea that nutrition isn't merely about physical health; it has profound implications for emotional and psychological well-being.

Dr. van der Kolk, in *The Body Keeps the Score*, emphasizes the connection between physical activity and mental health. He states, "Exercise is a powerful antidote to stress, anxiety, and depression."[17] Engaging in regular physical activity not only promotes physical health but also releases endorphins, which can enhance mood and alleviate feelings of distress. For those recovering from childhood trauma, exercise serves as a practical tool for managing symptoms and fostering a sense of agency and control over one's body and experiences. Furthermore, the physical act of moving and engaging with one's body can help survivors reconnect with themselves, fostering a sense of safety and stability that may have been lost during their traumatic experiences.

In her book *The Deepest Well*, Dr. Nadine Burke Harris wrote about exercise and nutrition at her clinic:

> *"We saw that exercising made a huge difference for our kids, but so did eating right. Making a few specific changes to what grade of fuel went in the tank (e.g., substituting lean proteins and complex carbohydrates for greasy fast food) improved the body's ability to regulate itself. We explained that exercising*

and eating healthfully not only contributed to weight loss but also helped boost the immune system and improve brain function.

We've talked about how inflammation is one of the ways a well-regulated immune system fights infection, but as with everything else in the body, balance is critical. Too much inflammation causes all sorts of problems, from digestive issues to cardiovascular complications. Eating foods that are high in omega-3 fatty acids, antioxidants, and the fiber from fruits, vegetables, and whole grains helps fight inflammation and bring the immune system back into balance. By contrast, a diet high in refined sugar, starches, and saturated fats can promote further inflammation and imbalance. By choosing a healthier pattern of eating and adding moderate exercise to their routines, sufferers have two great ways to bring their biological systems into better balance."[109]

Building on this idea, it's essential to explore specific dietary approaches that have garnered attention for their potential benefits in healing both mental and metabolic illnesses. One such approach is the ketogenic diet, which has been studied for its unique methods of optimizing health by making significant shifts in how our bodies convert food into energy.

The ketogenic diet, often referred to as the keto diet, emphasizes a high-protein, high-fat, low-carbohydrate intake that puts the body into a state of ketosis. In this state, the body becomes highly efficient at burning fat for fuel instead of relying on glucose from carbohydrates.

This shift not only aids weight management but also appears to have clear implications for mental and metabolic health.

Research suggests that ketogenic diets may offer neuroprotective effects, which can be especially beneficial for individuals struggling with conditions such as epilepsy, anxiety, and depression. By reducing the availability of glucose, the brain becomes more reliant on ketones, which are known to have stabilizing effects on neuronal activity. The result? Enhanced mood regulation and sharper cognitive function.

In addition, the keto diet has been linked to reduced inflammation, a key factor in many chronic conditions. By minimizing sugar intake and eliminating refined carbohydrates that trigger inflammatory responses, individuals can experience a decrease in symptoms related to both metabolic syndromes and mood disorders. The emphasis on healthy fats, particularly those rich in omega-3 fatty acids, further helps to combat inflammation, supporting optimal brain health.

Incorporating a keto lifestyle can lead to improved insulin sensitivity and balance in blood sugar levels, which are crucial in preventing and managing metabolic illnesses such as diabetes. The stabilization of these levels can have a domino effect, improving energy, reducing cravings, and promoting a more balanced mood—creating a positive feedback loop for those on their healing journey.

It's important to acknowledge the complexities of significant dietary changes, especially for those grappling with the lingering effects of childhood trauma, who often find solace in comfort foods as a form of emotional first aid. Moreover, the challenges of access and cost associated with high-protein, high-fat, low-carb diets can feel daunting. Often, the journey toward healthier eating is fraught with its own obstacles that extend beyond simple choice.

Just as Dr. Burke emphasizes the importance of a nutritious diet in fostering overall health, the ketogenic diet emerges as a compelling option for those looking to address both mental and metabolic health challenges. When we prioritize food as medicine, we not only empower our bodies but also nurture our minds.

The integration of healthy sleep, nutrition, and exercise creates a powerful triad that can significantly enhance the recovery process for individuals affected by childhood trauma. Dr. Schiraldi, Dr. Palmer, Dr. Burke and Dr. van der Kolk collectively underscore that self-care is not a luxury; it is a necessity.

As the insights from these respected authors illustrate, the journey toward recovery is not solely about addressing past pain; it is also about fostering a sustainable future filled with health, vitality, and resilience. Investing time and effort into the intentional practice of self-care not only prepares individuals for the healing journey but also builds a resilient framework that supports their ongoing recovery.

Known Healing Elements, Therapies, & Interventions

In this section, I will attempt to loosely categorize various elements, therapies, and interventions based on the severity of different disorders thought to be caused by childhood trauma. Please note that this list is not exhaustive or definitive; it reflects my limited knowledge and understanding of healing approaches that I believe to hold promise. Included in this compilation are both widely recognized and well-established methods, as well as lesser-known interventions that show potential for positive outcomes.

I emphasize that this information should not be construed as recommendations. Instead, view these items as possibilities worth exploring, allowing you to take an active role in your own investigation and decision-making process. Your unique journey deserves thoughtful consideration as you seek what resonates with your healing path.

Amid the overwhelming darkness of childhood trauma lies a flicker of hope—a call to action. Recognizing the scars of trauma as urgent and significant, we can advocate for the understanding, compassion, and healing necessary to break the patterns of suffering that plague our communities. By facing this harsh reality, we empower ourselves to be agents of change for ourselves and our loved ones.

Healing begins when we illuminate the shadows of adversity, transforming silence into dialogue, despair into solidarity, and trauma into resilience. In acknowledging the destruction wreaked by childhood trauma, we pave the way toward both personal and communal restoration—a collective rebirth where recovery is possible, and hope is reborn.

As we explore the pathways toward healing and redemption, let us carry forward the understanding that, while trauma may shape our existence, it does not have to define it.

Love & Connectiveness

For individuals grappling with the scars of childhood trauma, having a trusted person to turn to is not just beneficial; it is essential. The ability to feel safe and supported in relationships lays the foundation for healing and growth, bridging the disconnection that often accompanies trauma. This safe connection creates a space where individuals can feel they can share their experiences, confront their emotions, and reclaim their sense of self.

Humans are relational. Research consistently underscores that meaningful relationships are crucial to our well-being, as love and support from others serve as powerful catalysts for healing. Without this critical support, those who have endured childhood trauma may find themselves in a state of perpetual isolation, distanced from family, friends, and their own emotional world, which can hinder their journey toward recovery and fulfillment. In the delicate process of healing, having someone to confide in can transform moments of despair into opportunities for connection, understanding, and resilience.

Toxic stress can affect anyone, especially during childhood when coping skills are still being developed and the brain is maturing. This vulnerability is often exacerbated by the absence of a protective care-giver. However, there is significant reason for optimism. The impacts of toxic stress can be greatly diminished—even years later. Our brains are adaptable and can be rewired, allowing hidden emotional wounds to heal when we approach them with understanding, compassion, and effective strategies. Many of these approaches help regulate the stress response, positively influence our genetic expression, and protect our cellular structures. Furthermore, they can reshape detrimental patterns established by adverse childhood experiences (ACEs) and transform how we perceive ourselves.

What facilitates the healing of a traumatized brain? We've all heard the adage "time heals all wounds." However, the answer is not merely the passage of time, but the presence of mature love. This love—often expressed through care, respect, acceptance, compassion, and kind-ness—has a profound impact on both the brain and body. Love has the ability to soften traumatic memories and help us endure periods of suffering.

As renowned neuroscientist Dr. Richard Davidson emphasized, "It all comes down to love."

In his groundbreaking book, *The Adverse Childhood Experiences Recovery Workbook*, Dr. Glenn Schiraldi wrote the following about the need to "open up" and connect:

"We are indeed as sick as our secrets. It is not healthy to keep painful secrets bottled up inside. The road to healing and resilience-building starts with awareness. It is therapeutic to simply understand what is causing your pain and why. And having a constructive outlet for painful secrets furthers the healing journey. Most people find it somewhat curative to simply talk about their ACEs with a caring person. Many health professionals now advocate routine screening for ACEs as part of medical intakes, just as we assess weight and blood pressure.

In a large study, doctors asked patients to tell them how the ACEs that they'd reported on a screening tool had impacted them later in life. The patients said they felt accepted as doctors really listened to their deepest secrets and still wanted to see them again. Their stress of secret-keeping was reduced. Screening for ACEs in this way resulted in a 35% drop in doctor visits and an 11% drop in emergency room visits." 9

As we conclude this journey of understanding the profound impact of love and human connections in healing from childhood trauma, I want to encourage you to take a meaningful step forward in the event you are suffering in any way from childhood trauma. Remember, you don't have to walk this path alone. Seek someone you trust—whether it's a friend, family member, or a mental health professional—who can provide a supportive ear and a comforting presence. Opening up and sharing your story is not just a brave act; it is an essential part of the healing process.

Harnessing the power of connection can help lighten the burden of your past, transforming secrets into opportunities for understanding and growth. You deserve to be heard, validated, and surrounded by love. Reach out, lean into vulnerability, and allow the warmth of trusted relationships to guide you toward recovery and fulfillment. Healing is not only possible; it is a journey that is best embarked upon together with those who care for you. Remember, love is a powerful force. Let it be your ally as you reclaim your narrative and embrace the path ahead.

A Gift of Love & Connection

When I started dating my wife, Emilie, I opened up to her about my childhood memories—stories that would later find their way into my book, *The Kite That Couldn't Fly*. She listened attentively as I recounted the moments that had shaped me. One story stands out: my experience trying out for Little League baseball.

I had always loved the game. The crisp white uniforms, the snap of a new baseball cap, the thrill of a home run—it all captivated me. As soon as I was old enough, I eagerly anticipated the day I would try out for the team. But when that spring day finally arrived, it quickly turned into a moment of humiliation.

I excelled during the hitting tryouts. Growing up, I had played half-ball with my friends in the streets; it was a challenging game that required precision and skill, and I had mastered it with a broomstick and half a ball. In contrast, hitting a hardball with a hefty bat felt like a breeze.

But then came the fielding tryouts, and that's where my troubles began. I had no baseball glove. I had assumed, wrongly, that the coaches would provide them alongside the bats and balls. As I stood there, bare-handed, I felt the weight of my inexperience. I still recall the way the coaches chuckled as I struggled to field the ground balls without a glove. I failed to catch a single one, but caught every pop-up that soared into the air. The laughter echoed in my ears, and I walked away without a spot on the team.

Fast forward to my first birthday with Emilie, the day I turned 60. She surprised me with a gift that spoke of love and understanding: a beautiful Rawlings leather baseball glove. In that moment, I realized just how much I had longed for a glove all those years. It was not just a piece of equipment; it was the embodiment of a dream I had carried with me for half a century.

Emilie saw the child in me that still yearned for that connection to the game I once loved. As I held the glove in my hands and felt the supple leather, I was filled with gratitude for her thoughtfulness. She had given me more than just a gift; she made me feel seen, loved, and understood. This is just one example of how love heals.

Beauty: The Heart's Medicine

The philosophy that would later guide my understanding of healing didn't come from textbooks or therapists—it came from an ancient Frenchwoman who lived in our cramped house on May Avenue, speaking wisdom in a language I couldn't understand but somehow absorbed into my bones.

My *arrière-grand-mère*—my great-grandmother—was a study in contradictions. Small and fierce, with steel-gray hair pulled into a tight bun and eyes that seemed to hold the weight of two continents, she had crossed an ocean to give her family a better life. She refused to let us grandchildren speak French, determined that we would be fully American, free from the discrimination she'd witnessed against immigrants in Kankakee. The Polish were "polocks," the Italians were "wops," and the French were "frogs"—she wanted no part of that shame for us.

But her philosophy? That she shared freely, filtered through my grandmother Myrtle's colorful translations.

Mémère—my grandmother—was *arrière-grand-mère's* opposite in every way except love. Where Great-grandmother was serious and scholarly, Grandma was a walking comedy show. Her rear end was so enormous that she waddled when she walked, the back hem of her house dress perpetually hiking up, creating a dress that swooped low in front and high in back like a mismatched curtain. She was absolutely obsessed with passing gas and treated each eruption like a performance, gathering an audience before releasing what sounded like Gabriel's trumpet.

"Better out than in!" she'd announce with theatrical flair, or my personal favorite: she'd wave her giant house dress like a matador's cape and tell us kids to "catch it and paint it green!"

It was Grandma Myrtle who told us she wanted to march down to the courthouse and change her name because "Myrtle sounds like a fart in a bottle." The woman was gloriously inappropriate, and I suspect I inherited every ounce of it.

But when *arrière-grand-mère* held court in our tiny living room, surrounded by her stack of French books from the library, even Myrtle would settle down to translate those sacred lessons. The house would smell of coffee grounds and whatever magical gravy Grandma was simmering—she could put that French gravy on anything and make it delicious. I was Great-grandmother's favorite because I was the only grandchild who could hit a quail when hunting, and she loved nothing more than creamed quail on toast.

During these impromptu philosophy classes, *arrière-grand-mère* would speak with an intensity that made her seem angry, her weathered hands gesturing emphatically. But Grandma's translations always came wrapped in joy and laughter, as if she was delivering the same wisdom but through a completely different lens.

"*Arrière-grand-mère* says there are only two things in this world that can pierce the human heart," Myrtle would begin, settling her considerable frame into her chair. "Beauty and affliction. And she says—now listen good, children—the world is full of beauty, and beauty is the antidote to affliction."

The old woman would nod vigorously, then launch into what sounded like an impassioned lecture in rapid French.

"She's saying you've got to fill your heart with beauty, and it won't leave room for the bad stuff," Grandma would continue. "Beauty and love, they push out the pain. She wants you to look for it everywhere—in the trees outside that window, in a baby's face, in the way the sunset hits the kitchen wall."

Great-grandmother would then rattle off a long list in French—things she found beautiful—while Myrtle translated with increasing enthusiasm: "Flowers pushing through sidewalk cracks! The sound of rain on the roof! A perfectly ripe tomato! The way a bird's wing catches the light!"

My mother lived Great-grandmother's wisdom. During rainstorms, Mom would herd us all outside to splash and kick in the water rushing down the street gutters, always barefoot. As she splashed alongside us, she would sing with her operatic voice, her melody mixing with and in the key and the rhythm of rain on pavement. Here was a woman overworked and overwhelmed, never knowing where the next meal would come from, yet she saw beauty even in the storm. I recall asking her once as we stood soaked to the skin, "Won't we catch cold from being in the rain?"

She laughed, spinning in a puddle like a child, and called back over the thunder, "It's worth it!"

That was Mom—finding magic in the middle of chaos, teaching us that sometimes the most beautiful moments come disguised as ordinary rain.

I didn't understand then that my *arrière-grand-mère* was channeling the French philosopher Simone Weil, whose writings I wouldn't discover until college. But the seeds were planted in that cramped living room, with the smell of coffee and gravy and the sound of an old woman insisting that beauty was not luxury but necessity—medicine for wounded hearts.

Years later, when I studied philosophy formally, I recognized Weil's words immediately: "Beauty and affliction are the only two things that can pierce our hearts." My great-grandmother had been teaching us Simone Weil's philosophy decades before I knew the name, understanding instinctively that in a world full of trauma and pain, we must deliberately seek and create beauty as an act of survival.

When I think about healing from childhood trauma now, I understand what *arrière-grand-mère* was teaching us. Beauty isn't frivolous or optional—it's therapeutic. The deliberate practice of noticing beauty, of filling our vision with sunsets and flowers and kind faces, literally rewires our brains away from the frequency of fear and toward the frequency of hope.

This wisdom connects directly to another powerful healing practice that, like beauty, trains our minds to seek light in darkness—the transformative practice of gratitude.

Gratitude

Gratitude is not just a fleeting feeling; it is a powerful state of being that can significantly impact our emotional well-being and healing journey. For those who have experienced childhood trauma, cultivating an attitude of gratitude can be a critical component of recovery. By shifting our focus from what is lacking to what we do have, gratitude allows us to reclaim our power, foster resilience, and create a sense of abundance in our lives. This positive perspective can be a beacon of hope and healing, enabling us to process our past experiences and move forward with greater clarity and joy.

In my book, *The Kite That Couldn't Fly,* I explored this profound concept of gratitude through personal anecdotes from my childhood. One heartfelt story in particular demonstrates how gratitude can illuminate even the darkest moments. It reflects the lessons learned from my mother, who modeled gratitude as a way of life despite our challenging circumstances. Through her teachings, we embraced a mindset that champions appreciation over despair, demonstrating how this simple yet profound practice can transform our outlook on life.

As you read this excerpt, consider the weight of gratitude in your own healing journey and how it can serve as a guiding light through the hardships of trauma. Here is the chapter "We Have A Lightbulb" from *The Kite That Couldn't Fly.*

> "Gratitude is one of the strongest and most transformative
> states of being. It shifts your perspective from lack to
> abundance and allows you to focus on the good in your
> life, which in turn pulls more goodness into your reality."
> –Jen Sincero

It was 1956. The latest technology was a transistor radio with an earphone. Elvis had just released "Blue Suede Shoes." Eisenhower was president. It was such a different, simple time.

I grew up with a hierarchy of fears: no food, electricity, heat, water, and lowest on the ladder, no phone. Doing without was a way of life. It was inconvenient when services were turned off because the bill wasn't paid, but we always got by. In addition to the inconvenience and discomfort of going without, we also suffered embarrassment when others outside our home knew just how poor we were. The neighborhood kids could be cruel, so we did our best to fake it.

Our May Avenue home was tiny, only 900 square feet. The lighting was provided by a single pale light bulb hanging from the ceiling by a corded wire and an open socket with a pull chain. We couldn't purchase replacement light bulbs back then; the electric company provided them at no cost. You got an electric bill in the mail and paid it at designated hardware stores around town or the electric company. You received your light bulbs when you paid your bill, and the size of your bill determined the number of bulbs. The system worked. That is, if you had the money to pay your bill.

It was hard for Mom to make ends meet with Dad's small paychecks and so many mouths to feed. She was a master at juggling the bills, but most of the time, Mom was late paying the electric bill, and as a result, we were always short on light bulbs. Most of the time, we were down to one working light bulb at a time. I remember being without electricity, but I never remember a time when we didn't have at least one light bulb, which is impressive given the low life expectancy of light bulbs in the 1950s.

On this evening, like most evenings, we were all in the kitchen, with our one pale lightbulb burning in the center of the room. The house was heated by coal when we had it. When we didn't, Mom opened the lit oven, warming the downstairs nicely.

Bedtime was the ritual that signaled the end of the day. During the school year, the ceremony started with Mom baking the daily sheet cake, which was dessert for the next day's school lunches. It was made in a nine-inch by thirteen-inch pan, always from scratch. Just before we went to bed, she made the cake as the last act of the day. She tried to make it earlier in the day and hide it a few times, but somehow, she always made a second cake before bedtime. It is hard hiding a sweet-smelling cake from a bunch of children in a 900-square-foot home.

Mom's hands were always adorned with medical tape and, at times, even electrical tape, to cover the cracks in her hands from eczema. Mom was plagued with this skin disease from childhood until she was around 50 years old, when she outgrew it. She told us that we all had a cross to bear and that her cross was eczema.

Once the cake went into the oven, Mom made the frosting from milk, powdered sugar, butter, and vanilla extract. Mom played a game with us while mixing the frosting by asking, "What flavor icing would you like for tomorrow's lunch?"

We knew the options were chocolate, vanilla, cherry, strawberry, mint, or lemon. After everyone shouted out a different flavor, Mom took the vote. This evening, it was cherry. As we watched Mom take out her box of McCormick's food coloring, she stirred a few drops of red in the white icing. Magic—cherry icing! The power of imagination is incredible. It tasted like cherry. I still love cherry cake. This ritual brought us joy and hope because we would have cake for dessert the next day.

With the cake frosted and placed high on the refrigerator, Mom turned off the oven and shut the door. Silently, we drifted to the center of the room, under the lightbulb, waiting for Mom. She moved to the center of us, grasped the bottom of her threadbare apron, and pulled it up to grab and unscrew the hot lightbulb. Now, in the dark, with each of us gripping that apron, we shuffled over to the narrow stairs and ascended.

As we moved in the dark, Mom found different ways to say the same thing. "We have a lightbulb!" "Do you know how lucky we are to have a lightbulb?" "How many families don't have a light bulb?" "Thank you, Jesus, for our light bulb!" She continued until we reached the center of the attic floor, where she screwed our treasured pale light bulb into the socket, and once again, we had light.

Think how that situation could have played out. Maybe pity, anger, resentment, or depression for her and our circumstances. Not our mom; she was thankful for everything. She repeatedly taught this to her children. To this day, my siblings and I have an uncommon joy and thankfulness for everything.

This has always been my favorite May Avenue story to tell. If I'm going to tell a few stories to an audience, I begin with this story. It shines a light on some of my best memories as a child. The central message teaches a priceless lesson: gratitude and thankfulness are indispensable parts of happiness and well-being. The light bulb story is just one example of the hundred lessons Mom intuitively taught her children.

As it turns out, gratitude was our superpower.

Mom taught us gratitude by example and reinforced it with scripture: "Rejoice always, pray continually, give thanks in all circumstances; for this is God's will for you in Christ Jesus." 1 Thessalonians 5:16-18. Mom's favorite quote was "Our Lord loves a thankful heart."

In a book of Jewish ethical teachings, *Pirkei Avot*, there is a saying that translates to: "Who is the rich one? He who rejoices in his portions. Who rejoices in their portions? Those who are happy with what they have." Mom taught us to have a deep appreciation for everything we had and for life itself.

Mom worked hard at counteracting the pain of our deficiency. She acknowledged it could be good to have more, but that we already had enough. She taught us that no matter what was missing, there was always an abundance of things to be thankful for. Gratitude for what we did have became more profound when contrasted against the backdrop of unfulfilled desires.

Mom knew gratitude was valuable and correct, but did she know the gift she was giving her children? Did she know it would be a potent lifelong tool in our toolbox for happiness and fulfillment? Having this gift of gratitude, and after coming out the other side of the trauma, most of my siblings and I saw everything clearer, brighter, and more appealing. Coming into adult life with gratitude has given most Menards a heightened sense of joy, play, and a continual commitment to making the most of their lives. I can confidently say that I have squeezed every bit of joy I could out of my life.

Scientific evidence shows that gratitude can change brain function when practiced consistently and correctly, making us feel more content and joyful. In his groundbreaking book *The Neuroscience of Gratitude: Why Self-Help Has It All Wrong*, Andrew Humington compiled scientific data compelling that gratitude changes the brain's structure.

> *"The benefits span across all areas of your life—from the physical to the professional and even the spiritual—that are touched by the stress and anxiety of modern life. On a physiological level, gratitude can bolster your immune system, enhance your sleep quality, and reduce your pain and sensitivity. Professionally, a consistent practice of gratitude will leave you brimming with motivation, while your productivity soars and decision-making processes occur with ease and clarity. Spiritu-*

ally, gratitude deepens your sense of purpose and meaning and can finally uncover that piece of your life that has eluded you for so long. It empowers your personal compass that continually guides you toward personal growth and appreciation for your life and life in its entirety."[110]

Sound too good to be true? It's not.

Remember that the journey through trauma can be fraught with pain, but the practice of gratitude offers a pathway toward healing, connection, and joy.

Building Resilience

One of the most significant assets in the process of healing and recovery from childhood trauma is resilience—the ability to adapt, bounce back, and grow in the face of adversity. Building resilience not only aids in the recovery process but also empowers individuals to reclaim their lives and cultivate a sense of agency.

Resilience involves developing coping strategies that allow survivors of trauma to navigate their emotions and experiences more effectively. As individuals learn to understand and manage their feelings, they create a stable foundation for healing. This transformation can be facilitated through practices such as mindfulness, self-compassion, and building supportive relationships, all of which are essential elements of resilience.

In his book, *The Resilience Workbook*, Dr. Glenn Schiraldi emphasizes the importance of resilience in recovery. "Resilience is not just about bouncing back; it's about growing beyond."[111] This quote encapsulates the journey toward healing, highlighting that while individuals may face significant challenges, each step taken to build resilience can lead to growth and a renewed sense of purpose.

By fostering resilience, trauma survivors can reshape their narratives, shifting from victimhood to empowerment. They learn to recognize their strengths, find meaning in their experiences, and ultimately build a life rooted in hope rather than fear. Embracing resilience is not just a pathway to recovery; it is a crucial element in reclaiming one's identity and thriving in the aftermath of trauma.

As individuals invest in their resilience and commit to their healing journey, they pave the way for emotional well-being and a brighter future. Healing is possible, and resilience is a guiding light on that transformational path.

Trauma Therapy

Following is an excerpt from *The Adverse Childhood Experiences Recovery Workbook* by Dr. Glenn R. Schiraldi with some guidance on trauma therapy:

> *"As you undertake your healing journey, you might consider whether or not you wish to enlist the aid of a mental health professional, specifically a trauma therapist, to help you settle the aftereffects of ACEs. A skilled trauma therapist is like a coach or a guide. World-class athletes typically have a coach to provide perspective, to teach or reinforce needed skills, and to give moral support. A seasoned guide can help you get more out of a journey. Similarly, seeking a skilled mental health professional is like finding a coping coach or a guide to greater resilience. Seeking the right mental health professional is an act*

of wisdom that can speed recovery and alleviate needless suffering. You don't have to suffer needlessly for decades, because trauma specialists are discovering every year more and more effective ways to heal hidden wounds.

The natural tendency is to avoid painful memories. We do this by numbing emotions, denying that the past still hurts, or covering the pain through addictions (drugs, gambling, shopping, work, and so forth). However, avoidance leaves the memories untouched and likely to intrude into awareness in uncomfortable ways. The goal of therapy is to bring the "memory forward," neutralize its distressing aspects, and put the memory fragments together. Then the traumatic memory can be stored like one memory alongside the other memories in the file cabinet, not the only memory sitting on the desktop.

You might feel comfortable trying the skills in this workbook on your own. Or you might decide to find a therapist who can support you as you master these skills and deal with particularly distressing memories or symptoms. The remainder of this chapter will help you determine whether a trauma therapist might be right for you."[9]

Does Therapy Work?

Yes, it does. Good therapy can lessen trauma symptoms and lift self-esteem. For example, trauma therapy for sexually abused children and adolescents has been found to improve self-esteem.[112] Therapy changes gene expression resulting in a calmer brain.[113]

Quite often, trauma survivors "fear that they are damaged to the core and beyond redemption."[17] Perhaps an unsuccessful experience with a psychotherapist in the past led you to believe that nothing can help. However, my experience tells me that there is no hole so deep or dark that one cannot climb out of it, especially with the right help. Again, love—along with calm and safety—is the healing agent.

Mature love replaces fear and binds hidden wounds. As Lewis and colleagues stated, "Love is not only an end for therapy; it is also the means whereby every end is reached."[114] And what is true for surgery is true for therapy. "Only human love keeps this from being the act of two madmen."[115]

When to Consider Therapy

You might seriously consider therapy if you are still suffering and struggling. Sometimes self-care and time cannot provide sufficient relief. Perhaps your symptoms have even worsened over time. If you're unsure whether therapy might help, ask yourself if any of the following symptoms sound familiar, and know that therapy can help address them all.

- You can't think of certain memories without intense distress.

- You experience memory intrusions, including nightmares, flashbacks, or hallucinations.

- You or your surroundings seem unreal.

- You drift away mentally during stressful times.

- You experience disturbing emotions on a frequent or chronic basis. These can include crushing feelings of low self-worth, shame, guilt, fear, depression, irritability, or extreme anger. Being negative or harshly self-critical can reflect unresolved inner pain.

- You feel numb, unable to experience happy feelings.

- You have a mental illness, such as anxiety, panic disorder, depression, or bipolar disorder, that willpower alone is not helping.

- You are harming or are about to harm yourself. (For example, cutting or otherwise injuring your body; having suicidal thoughts or behaviors; not taking care of yourself, such as avoiding needed medical care; having poor sleep, eating, or exercise habits; or having unprotected sex; engaging in risky behaviors such as driving dangerously or while intoxicated.)

- You have an addiction—such as to drugs, alcohol, gambling, eating, or work—along with trauma symptoms. (Look for a therapist who can treat the addiction as you process traumatic memories.)

- You can't function at home or on the job. (For example, you have trouble concentrating or doing simple tasks; you avoid people or places you need to be.)

- Stress interferes with your sleep; you have excessive daytime fatigue.

- Your relationships are being harmed by patterns formed earlier in life.

- You sense that something from the past might be damaging your mental or physical health.

- Any memories or symptoms seem overwhelming.

Seeking therapy for childhood trauma is not a sign of weakness but rather an act of courage and wisdom. Just as a skilled guide can help navigate treacherous terrain, a qualified trauma therapist can illuminate the path toward healing. While self-help resources like what is included in this book provide valuable tools, professional support may be crucial for processing deeper wounds and reconstructing fragmented memories.

Remember, there is no hole so deep that you cannot climb out of it with the right help. Whether you choose to work through trauma independently or with professional guidance, the key is to move forward with patience, self-compassion, and the understanding that healing is always possible.

Recalibrating Fragmented Traumatic Memories: Confronting the Past

Confronting the pain of our own experiences can be incredibly challenging, especially for those who have endured childhood trauma. Witnessing the suffering of others is difficult enough, so it's no surprise that survivors often struggle to face their own memories. To escape the overwhelming emotional turmoil, many may resort to numbing strategies like drugs, alcohol, or self-harm. However, when possible, it is essential for individuals to engage with and understand what has happened to them, even if this can be difficult—particularly for experiences predating conscious memory.

Trauma memories are frequently fragmented. When a traumatic event occurs, the intense stress and emotional upheaval can disrupt how those memories are encoded and stored in the brain. Rather than forming a coherent narrative, trauma memories can become disjointed, with some details vividly remembered while others are blurred or entirely missing. This fragmentation can lead to confusion, distress, and difficulty in processing the event.

Several factors contribute to the fragmentation of trauma memories. One significant factor is dissociation, a psychological defense mechanism that often occurs in response to overwhelming stress. This can result in a disconnection from thoughts, emotions, and even physical sensations during the traumatic experience. Additionally, the profound emotional impact of trauma can hinder a person's ability to integrate the experience fully, leading to memories that manifest more as sensory impressions—like images, sounds, or feelings—rather than a structured narrative. Neurobiological effects also play a role; traumatic experiences can impact brain regions involved in memory processing, such as the hippocampus and amygdala as discussed in Book One, which can further splinter and fragment memories.

Therapists who specialize in childhood trauma recovery often employ a range of techniques to help individuals make sense of, integrate, and recalibrate their trauma memories. Somatic Experiencing is one effective intervention that focuses on the individual's body sensations, helping to release stored tension linked to trauma. By tuning into these physical sensations, individuals can engage more fully with their memories. Narrative Therapy is another impactful approach, where therapists assist individuals in constructing coherent narratives about their traumatic experiences. This process allows survivors to reframe their stories, find meaning, and foster healing.

Reconstructing trauma memories can lead to several positive outcomes. First, it can significantly reduce emotional distress, allowing individuals to experience less pain and anxiety linked to those memories. Creating a coherent narrative also empowers survivors by providing them a sense of control and understanding over their experiences, which can facilitate moving forward. Furthermore, gaining a fuller understanding of traumatic memories enhances coping mechanisms and resilience when confronted with challenging emotions or triggers in the future.

In summary, recalibrating fragmented trauma memories can be profoundly beneficial, paving the way for healing and a healthier emotional state. If you or someone you know is navigating the complexities of trauma, seeking support from a qualified therapist can be a crucial step toward recovery.

Proven & Promising Trauma-Processing Treatments

In his landmark book, *The Body Keeps the Score*, Dr. van der Kolk gave an overview of how trauma recovery works:

"There are fundamentally three avenues:
1) top down, by talking, (re-)connecting with others, and allowing ourselves to know and understand what is going on with us, while processing the memories of the trauma;
2) by taking medicines that shut down inappropriate alarm reactions, or by utilizing other technologies that change the way the brain organizes information, and

3) bottom up: by allowing the body to have experiences that deeply and viscerally contradict the helplessness, rage, or collapse that result from trauma.

Which one of these is best for any particular survivor is an empirical question. Most people I have worked with require a combination."[17]

Relating your story in words and replacing unreasonably negative thoughts calm the arousal centers of the brain and help complete the healing process. However, trauma memories, which are situated in the visual, emotional, and survival brain regions, might initially be inaccessible to words and logic. Therefore, many of the effective treatment modalities do not rely primarily on words and logic. Rather, they access implicit memories with minimal or no verbalizing. The following list includes treatments that have delivered effective healing.

Body-Based Therapies

In this approach, the therapist helps bring the client back to optimal arousal levels, where stress levels are neither too high nor too low. In this window of tolerance, you are hardwired to talk calmly and logically, regulate emotions, and feel connected to your body. Storytelling takes a back seat to what is going on in your body. The therapist monitors subtle changes in your body and might say, "Let's put telling your story aside for a moment. It looks like your shoulders tense when you talk about that memory. Pay attention to that."

Simply tracking what is going on in the body helps calm physical and emotional arousal and restores a sense of connection to the self. Remember: Under excessive stress, the brain kicks into survival mode. In the urgency to fight or flee, areas of the brain concerned with logic, speech, and connection to the self go offline. Tracking these physical responses helps bring these areas back online.

The therapist might also say, "Think of a strength or other resource that helped you get through all that. Notice how your body feels as you think of it. How does that feel emotionally? Let that settle in your body." Or the therapist might suggest, "It seems like your body wants to complete an action that you weren't permitted to complete back then. I wonder what would happen if you planted your feet firmly on the ground and from the strength of your core slowly pushed back against the perpetrator." The client slowly completes the action impulse and tracks how that feels in the body. Now, action replaces the freezing state that was locked in the memory.

Such body-based approaches have been pioneered by Drs. Bessel van der Kolk (2014), Patricia Ogden (Ogden and Fisher 2015; sensorimotor psychotherapy), and Peter Levine (2010; somatic experiencing).

Cognitive Behavioral Analysis Systems of Psychotherapy (CBASP)

The Cognitive Behavioral Analysis System of Psychotherapy (CBASP), developed by James McCullough in 2000, is a pioneering integrative therapeutic approach designed specifically for chronically depressed adults. Recognizing that individuals with chronic depression often feel a deep sense of disconnection from their environments, CBASP seeks to bridge this gap by enhancing access to vital feedback regarding problematic interpersonal dynamics and relationships.

Central to CBASP is the idea that this disconnection hinders individuals from recognizing how their behaviors impact others, perpetuating a cycle of isolation and emotional distress. By leveraging the therapeutic relationship, CBASP fosters an environment where patients can cultivate empathy, gain insight into their interpersonal patterns, and confront and heal from past interpersonal trauma.

CBASP utilizes three core techniques to support this process:

1. **Situational Analysis:** This problem-solving technique empowers patients to understand the consequences of their behaviors on others, encouraging them to modify maladaptive interactions in real time.
2. **Interpersonal Discrimination Exercises:** Through this examination, patients reflect on past traumatic experiences to differentiate between unhealthy and healthier relationships, thereby refining their understanding of social dynamics and improving their relational interactions.
3. **Behavioral Skill Training/Rehearsal:** This component includes practical exercises, such as assertiveness training, aimed at equipping depressed individuals with the skills necessary to enact positive behavioral changes in their lives.

Overall, Cognitive Behavioral Analysis System of Psychotherapy stands out as a tailored therapy that not only addresses the symptoms of chronic depression but also promotes healing and growth through enhanced interpersonal skills, ultimately guiding individuals towards a more connected and fulfilling life.

Dialectical Behavioral Therapy (DBT)

Dialectical Behavioral Therapy (DBT), developed by Dr. Marsha Linehan in the late 1980s, is a specialized form of cognitive behavioral therapy designed to help individuals struggling with emotional dysregulation, self-destructive behaviors, and interpersonal issues. While originally created for individuals with borderline personality disorder,

DBT has proven effective for a range of emotional and behavioral challenges, including healing from childhood trauma.

At its core, DBT emphasizes the balance between acceptance and change, encapsulated in its name. "Dialectical" refers to the synthesis of opposites, such as acceptance of one's current situation while also striving for meaningful change. This dual focus fosters a compassionate approach that validates the experiences and feelings of individuals while encouraging them to develop healthier coping mechanisms.

DBT consists of four key components:

1. **Mindfulness:** This foundational skill teaches individuals to become more aware of their thoughts, emotions, and bodily sensations in the present moment. Mindfulness is particularly beneficial for trauma survivors, as it can help them stay grounded when experiencing overwhelming emotions or flashbacks.

2. **Distress Tolerance:** This module equips individuals with strategies to cope with crises and intense emotional pain without resorting to harmful behaviors. For those healing from childhood trauma, building distress tolerance skills is crucial in navigating triggers and managing urges to escape painful feelings.

3. **Emotion Regulation:** This component focuses on identifying, understanding, and regulating emotions. Individuals learn to recognize their emotional responses and develop strategies to manage them more effectively, decreasing the likelihood of becoming overwhelmed by traumatic memories or feelings.

4. **Interpersonal Effectiveness:** This aspect of DBT provides tools to improve communication and relationship-building skills. By learning to express needs and set boundaries assertively, trauma survivors can cultivate healthier connections and reduce patterns of isolation or conflict rooted in their past experiences.

Dialectical Behavioral Therapy's structured approach and emphasis on skill-building make it particularly suited for individuals healing from childhood trauma. By providing practical tools and fostering a sense of safety within the therapeutic environment, the principles of DBT empower individuals to process their trauma, rebuild their sense of self, and create fulfilling relationships.

Eye Movement Desensitization & Reprocessing (EMDR)

EMDR is a specialized therapy originally developed to help individuals process traumatic memories and reduce the distress associated with them. The approach involves guiding clients to recall distressing events while simultaneously engaging in bilateral stimulation, such as eye movements, taps, or sounds. This dual focus is believed to facilitate the brain's natural processing mechanisms, making it easier to integrate and heal from traumatic experiences.

Research has shown that EMDR can be particularly effective for those suffering from PTSD, anxiety, and depression. Clients often find that their emotional responses to traumatic memories are significantly reduced, allowing them to move forward in their lives with greater emotional resilience and stability.

Accelerated Resolution Therapy (ART)

Accelerated Resolution Therapy (ART) is a relatively new, evidence-based treatment designed to help individuals overcome traumatic memories in a brief, well-tolerated, and effective manner. Similar to EMDR, ART utilizes bilateral eye movements to aid in the reprocessing of memories, but it also incorporates guided imagery techniques.

Clients are encouraged to visualize their traumatic experiences and then transform them into positive outcomes or images.

This method can result in a rapid decrease in symptoms associated with PTSD, anxiety, and depression. ART emphasizes symptom relief and resolution, helping clients gain a sense of control over their thoughts and feelings while facilitating emotional healing. Research to date suggests that ART provides impressive results, often in fewer sessions than EMDR.

Instinctual Trauma Response (ITS)

This innovative therapeutic approach gently fast-tracks the healing process, neutralizing fear and stress, and providing a sense of structure and resolution to troubling trauma memories. The survivor draws ("The body remembers what the mind forgets") the trauma memory according to the six stages of the instinctual trauma response. The therapist posts the drawings and then compassionately recounts the story as the survivor, watching from a safe distance, realizes that the memory is now completed and in the past. The externalized dialogue between the survivor's true self and traumatized part(s) that contain stuck, dysfunctional thoughts and other reactions completes the healing process. ITR can be done virtually or in person. Properly trained caregivers can even guide their children through the ITR process.

Art Therapy

Art Therapy is a creative therapeutic approach that utilizes artistic expression as a means of promoting emotional healing and self-discovery. Through various art forms—such as painting, drawing, sculpture, and collage—clients are encouraged to express their thoughts, feelings, and experiences nonverbally. This can be particularly beneficial for individuals who find it challenging to articulate their emotions or trauma.

Art therapists use the creative process as a tool for reflection, exploration, and communication, allowing individuals to confront and process their feelings in a safe and supportive environment. Research has indicated that art therapy can help reduce symptoms of anxiety, depression, and trauma, fostering personal growth and healing through creativity.

Each of these therapeutic interventions offers unique methods and advantages, catering to the diverse needs of individuals seeking healing from trauma and emotional distress.

In Chapter 15, I recounted Trent's poignant journey—a man whose deep-seated childhood trauma came to light at the age of 50, manifesting as a host of debilitating mental disorders, the most harrowing being an acute sense of suicidality. In the throes of despair, Trent felt as though his mind was slipping away, unaware of the dark shadows of his past that had cast such a long and painful shadow over his life. It was only after considerable introspection and exploration that he uncovered the painful truth of severe abuse he endured as an infant at the hands of his mother. This revelation marked the beginning of Trent's arduous path toward healing, a journey he continues to navigate with determination and hope.

Stella Center

In his quest for understanding and respite, Trent discovered the transformative work being done at the Stella Center—an innovative interventional psychiatry practice dedicated to providing biological treatments tailored specifically for individuals grappling with the debilitating effects of childhood trauma. This groundbreaking center addresses the root causes of pervasive symptoms such as panic attacks, anxiety, sleep disturbances, and irritability, which often plague trauma survivors.

What sets the Stella Center apart is its revolutionary model of trauma treatments that brings forth rapid and effective relief—solutions that are anchored in rigorous research and modern science. Rather than merely offering a procedural fix or a transient infusion, Stella employs a meticulously curated approach to care that is personalized for each client, acknowledging the uniqueness of their experiences and needs. This holistic strategy is reshaping the landscape of post-traumatic stress treatment, ushering in a new era of mental healthcare and is proving a beacon of hope.

Trent's remarkable progress, along with the heartfelt testimonials from over 9,500 individuals treated across 20 locations nationwide, stands as a testament to the exceptional care offered by the Stella Center. Here, the focus is not on merely managing symptoms; rather, it is on truly healing the wounds of the past. As Trent continues to thrive under this compassionate care, it becomes increasingly clear that the Stella Center is at the forefront of a vital shift in mental health treatment, one that prioritizes comprehensive recovery and restores hope to those who have suffered in silence for far too long.

I've included a partial list of the interventions and therapies offered at the Stella Center.

Stellate Ganglion Block (SGB)

Stellate Ganglion Block (SGB) is a procedure in which a local anesthetic is injected next to the stellate ganglion, a collection of the sympathetic nerves located in the neck that helps regulate many involuntary functions such as heart rate, blood pressure and sweating. For years, Stellate Ganglion Block (SGB) has been recognized as an FDA-approved pain-relieving treatment. Most recently, Stellate Ganglion Block (SGB) has been used off-label to treat symptoms of PTSD, anxiety and depression because it helps regulate the brain's overactive sympathetic nervous system and "reset" the fight-or-flight response to its baseline.

After the SGB treatments, many patients have experienced: better sleep, better memory and concentration, decrease in anxiety, panic attacks and depression, an ability to connect with others again, less jumpiness or nervousness, and improved intimacy and sexual function.

Ketamine Infusion Therapy

Ketamine is a chemical that is FDA-approved as a dissociative anesthetic. It has also been researched for over 50 years as an antidepressant and now used as an off-label drug for the management of conditions like treatment-resistant depression, anxiety disorders, and post-traumatic stress disorder (PTSD).

It can provide rapid and life-transferring relief when other treatments don't work. Unlike traditional antidepressants (e.g., SSRIs, SNRIs) that primarily affect serotonin, norepinephrine, and dopamine levels, ketamine works by blocking the NMDA receptor in the brain and interacting with brain neurotransmitters. By increasing the levels of glutamate in the brain, ketamine can strengthen neural communication as well as repair the damage caused by cortisol and other stress hormones. As a result, new insights and thought patterns can emerge and replace the negative thought patterns that kept individuals stuck in the cycle of depression.

In an intravenous (IV) infusion, ketamine is delivered directly into the bloodstream through a small needle placed in a vein in your arm. It is considered as the "gold standard" of delivering ketamine due to efficacy and the easiness to control and adjust the dose based on the patients' history and on-site reactions. Compared to other delivery methods, IV ketamine administers medication in a safer and more precise manner, and can take effect at a predictable time.

Spravato Treatment

Spravato® is a treatment that provides transformative relief from depression symptoms. In a Spravato® therapy, a nasal spray form of esketamine (half molecule of ketamine) is administered by certified clinical staff. Currently, it is the only FDA-approved ketamine therapy accessible to patients and is covered by most insurances. It has shown to be one of the most promising modalities for treatment-resistant depression (TRD) in patients with major depressive disorder (MDD) with suicidal thoughts or actions.

Unlike traditional antidepressants (e.g., SSRIs, SNRIs) that primarily affect serotonin, norepinephrine, and dopamine levels, esketamine works by blocking the NMDA receptor in the brain, resulting in an increase in neural connections, effectively rewiring circuits in the brain and helping patients form new and more positive patterns of thinking.

Transcranial Magnetic Stimulation (TMS) Treatment

TMS is an FDA-cleared, non-invasive treatment that uses magnetic fields to stimulate nerve cells in the brain. It is proven to improve symptoms of major depressive disorder by sending magnetic pulses that regulate activity in the neural circuits in the prefrontal cortex, the region of the brain most consistently impaired by depression. Research on TMS therapy's efficacy for depression can be dated as early as the 1980s. Transcranial magnetic stimulation (TMS) is a biological treatment for depression that's rooted in brain science. Newer studies have found that

TMS therapy also showed promise in treating other mental challenges like OCD and PTSD.

After TMS treatments, many patients have experienced: improved mood, increased energy levels, better sleep, enhanced cognitive function, pain relief, and reduced anxiety.

Psychedelic-Assisted Therapy

Recent research has shown that certain psychedelic substances, such as psilocybin (found in magic mushrooms) and MDMA, can facilitate therapeutic breakthroughs in processing trauma. When used in conjunction with psychotherapy, these substances may help individuals confront and integrate painful memories, enhance emotional connection, and foster a sense of well-being. Clinical trials have reported promising outcomes for PTSD, depression, and anxiety when integrating psychedelics into a structured therapeutic framework.

While there is clearly growing interest and research supporting the use of psychedelics in therapy, commercial availability is currently limited and primarily focused on ketamine. As research continues and regulatory frameworks develop, it is likely that more options for psychedelic-assisted therapy will become widely accessible in the future. However, patients should stay informed about the legal and clinical landscape in their area and consult licensed health professionals for guidance.

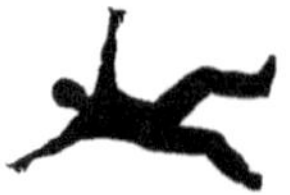

The journey from trauma to healing requires patience, compassion, and unwavering commitment. Recovery is built on a foundation of essential self-care—prioritizing sleep, proper nutrition, and physical movement that helps trauma survivors reconnect with their bodies. From there, a spectrum of therapeutic interventions awaits, from EMDR and CBT to innovative treatments like those offered at the Stella Center. Each individual's path is unique; what proves effective for one person may not work for another. Survivors must be willing to explore different approaches and pivot when necessary.

Progress is rarely linear. There will be setbacks and days when patients feel they've slipped backward on the numerical scale we discussed earlier. But healing is measured not in the absence of difficult days, but in one's growing capacity to navigate them with resilience. Every incremental movement toward zero and beyond deserves recognition. No one walks this path alone—thousands have journeyed toward healing before, and thousands more are on that same journey today.

The shadows of the past do not have to dictate the future. With the right tools, support, and determination, individuals can move from merely surviving to truly living. The work of reclaiming one's life is among the bravest endeavors a person can undertake.

CHAPTER TWENTY-ONE

The Deep Root Cure

"No tree, it is said, can grow to heaven unless its roots reach down to hell."

–Carl Jung

Tree House Recovery: A Model of Multidimensional Healing

IN MY SEARCH FOR effective approaches to healing childhood trauma, I discovered an organization that stands as a beacon of innovation in the addiction recovery landscape—Tree House Recovery. Their success rates in achieving sustained sobriety are remarkable, especially when compared to conventional treatment models. What makes their approach particularly significant for this book is not merely their effectiveness in treating addiction, but their profound understanding of the complex interplay between childhood trauma, neurobiological development, and addictive behaviors.

A Vision Born from Lived Experience

Tree House Recovery began with Justin McMillen, a man whose personal journey through addiction and recovery illuminates the transformative potential that lies within even the darkest human experiences. By age 30, Justin had reached what he describes as a profound surrender—not the hopeful surrender often romanticized in recovery circles, but a bleak acceptance that his life would end in that garage where he was squatting, surrounded by the detritus of addiction.

"It's beyond a loss of a will to live," Justin explained to me. "It's just, 'Oh, okay. This is who I am. I am the worst of what anyone could have imagined that I am.'"

Yet from this desolate place emerged an extraordinary transformation. Through a series of events that brought people into his life who served as both mirrors reflecting his current state and windows into what he could become, Justin found his way to sobriety. But unlike many who are content to focus solely on their personal recovery, Justin felt compelled to bring others with him on this journey of healing.

"It's never been enough for me just to get sober," he shared. "I had to bring the whole damn world with me."

This passionate vision evolved into Tree House Recovery, an organization that approaches addiction not as a moral failing or a simple disease, but as a complex, multidimensional challenge requiring an equally sophisticated response.

The Undeniable Connection: Childhood Trauma & Addiction

One of the most striking revelations from my conversations with Tree House Recovery staff is the overwhelming prevalence of childhood trauma among their clients. When I asked Mary Dowd, Clinical Supervisor at their North Carolina location, what percentage of their clients have experienced childhood trauma, her response was immediate: "I would say 95%."

This figure was consistently echoed by other staff members. Robert Mo, Clinical Director at their Orange County location and notably the first person to go through the Tree House program, confirmed this assessment. When asked the same question, he stated unequivocally: "100%."

George Coleman, developer of their "Naked Writing" program, went even further, suggesting that "95% have experienced childhood trauma, and the other 5% are lying," he said half-jokingly.

This perspective was confirmed yet again in my conversation with Neal Trusso, the first Physical Empowerment Director at Tree House. When posed the same question, Neal reported: "I would say easily, over 80%." He went on to describe how, during his 90-day reviews with clients at Tree House, "about 95% of the guys that I interviewed all said something between the ages of 13 and 15 happened and they chose drugs." This striking pattern suggests critical developmental windows when trauma manifests as behavioral choices.

These consistent observations from experienced clinicians point to an inescapable conclusion: the relationship between childhood trauma and addiction is not merely correlational but fundamental. As Mary explained, "When you interview a client, I already know there's going to be abuse in there—maybe physical, neglect, sexual, whatever. I know that there's some aspect of that, pretty much for everybody...varying degrees, but it's there."

Understanding the Outliers: When Trauma Isn't Obvious

My conversation with Brent Botros, who runs the Tree House program in Wilmington, North Carolina, offered a fascinating counterpoint to this pattern. Brent described himself as "an outlier" with "a perfect zero" on his ACE score. His childhood, by conventional measures, was secure and privileged:

"I was kind of given everything on a silver platter... I think I only remember one time during my childhood my parents getting into a heated argument, and it didn't even last that long."

Yet Brent's journey into addiction began in high school and spiraled dramatically over the years, eventually leading to homelessness, criminal activity, and near-death experiences. How does this square with the trauma-addiction connection?

Digging deeper, Brent revealed that his mother had experienced significant childhood trauma, including sexual and physical abuse. This points to what researchers call epigenetics—the way trauma can affect gene expression across generations. Additionally, Brent described himself as having "always had this feeling like something was a little bit different with me" and being "always an adrenaline junkie."

As he put it: "Even though I came from, like, a pretty secure environment growing up there were still a lot of times where I kind of felt over-sheltered and like I had to break away from that and stir the pot and make things chaotic. So, it was almost like I craved a level of chaos that I never had when I was a kid."

This suggests that even in the absence of overt trauma, certain neurobiological predispositions—perhaps inherited epigenetically from his mother's trauma—created vulnerability to addiction. This aligns with Justin's theory about genetic "warriors" and "worriers" whose neurobiological makeup may make them more susceptible to addiction in modern environments.

The Warrior & the Worrier: Genetic Foundations of Vulnerability

Tree House Recovery's most compelling insights relate to the genetic predispositions that may influence vulnerability to addiction. Justin proposes that certain genetic traits—particularly those affecting the dopaminergic system—create a predisposition that can lead to either exceptional achievement or addiction.

"I believe that a predisposition to addiction is the exact same thing as a predisposition to high performance through most of human history," Justin told me. "I think that those of us who are 'addicts' are simply part of the species that's dying off. Modernity is wiping us out."

This perspective frames addiction not as a defect but as a mismatch between evolutionary adaptations and modern environments. Traits that were once survival advantages—novelty-seeking, high drive, hypersensitivity to environmental inputs—may now create vulnerability in a world that requires different adaptations.

Justin's team is working with geneticists to explore this theory, focusing particularly on two genetic profiles they've observed among people with addiction:

1. **The Warrior**: Characterized by novelty-seeking behavior, high drive, and an inability to be satisfied. These individuals constantly seek "more" and may struggle with the sedentary nature of modern life.
2. **The Worrier**: Distinguished by rumination, racing thoughts, and hypersensitivity to environmental inputs. These individuals process

stimuli more intensely than others, potentially making them more vulnerable to trauma's impacts.

Both profiles share a common thread: difficulty with dopamine regulation. Research suggests that individuals predisposed to addiction may have issues with dopamine reuptake or may metabolize dopamine more quickly than others, creating a neurochemical drive for substances or behaviors that temporarily regulate their system.

The Three-Dimensional Approach to Recovery

What distinguishes Tree House Recovery's approach is their recognition that addiction cannot be reduced to a single cause or treated through a one-dimensional solution. Instead, they view human beings as systems comprised of three interdependent dimensions:

1. **Biological (Hardware)**: The physical structure, including our genetics, brain chemistry, and physiological responses.
2. **Psychological (Software)**: Our thoughts, beliefs, emotions, and the mental frameworks through which we interpret the world.
3. **Social (Network)**: The relationships, environments, and connections that provide inputs to our system.

These dimensions are not isolated but deeply interconnected—a change in one inevitably affects the others. As Justin explained, "To say what fundamentally causes addiction is the same as someone saying what causes a computer to malfunction. It's never going to be just one thing... it's likely going to be a combination."

Robert Mo summarized this approach as "biopsychosocial spiritual"—a comprehensive framework that addresses all aspects of a person's experience. This holistic approach is what sets Tree House apart from other programs, according to Mary: "I see a difference with Tree House than any other program I've ever worked with."

The Healing Power of Movement: A Neurobiological Necessity

A cornerstone of Tree House Recovery's approach is their emphasis on physical movement as essential to healing. Neal Trusso, who developed their physical empowerment program, explained that they "firmly believed that physical activity in a very structured, purposeful way would help heal the body and brain faster."

This isn't merely about exercise as a healthy habit; it's about addressing a fundamental neurobiological need. As Justin explained, "Dopamine is also the movement molecule. Some of us just simply have to move more, and it's about keeping the brain healthy. If our brain is not healthy, our neurochemistry is not healthy."

Neal pointed to scientific validation of this approach: "After meeting with one of the Harvard professors, [we learned that] any type of work you do physically, like working out in any way, it actually worked your brain out too. So brains were getting healthier faster."

The Harvard professor Neal referenced is Dr. John Ratey, author of the groundbreaking book *Spark: The Revolutionary New Science of Exercise and the Brain*. Dr. Ratey's research demonstrates that exercise isn't just beneficial for physical health—it fundamentally changes brain chemistry in ways that enhance learning, attention, self-confidence, and emotional regulation.[116]

This scientific perspective transforms how we understand the relationship between movement and mental health. As Dr. Ratey writes in *Spark*:

> *"Exercise is the single most powerful tool you have to optimize your brain function... exercise strengthens the cellular machinery of learning. BDNF [Brain-Derived Neurotrophic Factor] improves the function of neurons, encourages their growth, and strengthens and protects them against the natural process of cell death. It's like fertilizer for the brain."*[116]

For individuals with dopaminergic system differences, movement is not optional—it's essential for proper brain function. Without adequate physical activity, these individuals may struggle with focus, emotional regulation, and overwhelming internal discomfort. Tree House Recovery's approach recognizes that for many people with addiction—especially those with ADD/ADHD traits—the sedentary nature of modern life creates a neurochemical deficit that substances temporarily fill.

Neal emphasized that this physical component serves multiple purposes: "We could get guys to push themselves. We could force better sleeping and eating habits earlier in recovery and basically supercharge things... so we could work on anxiety, PTSD, self-esteem, all those things through the physical side."

This reflects my own research findings about the three pillars of mental health: movement, nutrition, and sleep. As I shared with Neal: "Dr. Palmer [author of 'Brain Energy']... has a belief that this whole disruption, addiction, all the disorders that come from trauma, it starts at the cellular level... And his bottom line is, there are three things that will lead to optimum mental health and will overcome disorders in the mind, including mental illness: movement, nutrition, and sleep."

The transformation is visible in their clients' physicality—many develop athletic physiques that reflect not vanity but neurochemical optimization. As Brandon, a staff member, told me when I visited the Nashville facility: "Brother, I need you out on this floor. I can get you to an optimal fitness level that'll start the good chemicals flowing in your brain."

Beyond Physical Movement: The Healing Power of Creative Expression

Neal added an important dimension to our understanding of "movement" that extends beyond physical exercise: "It doesn't necessarily mean working out in the gym... my son is a guitarist at [a university in] Nashville now... and we talk about this. Reading, playing, and performing music actuates those parts of your brain too. So it's music, it's singing, it's art, it's everything."

This insight connects to my own experience with music as a healing modality. As I shared with Neal: "I'm the only of only one of 14 that had classical music training. I started at age six, and I've been taking it ever since. And I am different, not better, just different. I'm creative. I have 14 patents. I have more energy. I'm 74. I'm not losing cognition yet."

This expanded understanding of "movement" reminds us that healing can come through many forms of active engagement—whether physical exercise, creative expression, or other forms of meaningful activity that stimulate the brain in healthful ways.

Naked Writing: Bringing Light to Darkness

Among Tree House Recovery's most powerful interventions is a process called "Naked Writing," developed by George Coleman, a Vietnam veteran who discovered the healing potential of journaling through his own journey with PTSD.

George explained to me that we all have an "internal curtain" behind which we hide the thoughts, memories, and emotions that feel too painful or shameful to acknowledge. Naked Writing is the practice of putting these hidden aspects of ourselves onto paper—dragging them from behind the curtain into the light where they can be acknowledged and processed.

As Robert Mo, who oversees the Naked Writing program at the Orange County location, explained, this process creates a safe context for vulnerability, allowing clients to externalize their internal pain.

I found this approach particularly resonant because my own healing journey began with a similar process. Writing *The Kite That Couldn't Fly* allowed me to revisit and process childhood memories I had long buried. As I wrote, my 12-year-old self became my guide through the tiny May Avenue house where I grew up, showing me scenes I had tucked away behind my own internal curtain.

The therapeutic value of this process was profound. Discussing these memories with my siblings, especially my brother Jamie, allowed us to confirm their reality and make sense of them together. Some stories were too painful to include in my published memoir, but the act of writing them down and speaking about them was transformative. As I told George, "A heavy weight has been lifted. No more boogie men behind my curtain."

EMDR: Transformative Healing for Deep Trauma

In my conversation with Mary Dowd, who specializes in EMDR (Eye Movement Desensitization and Reprocessing) therapy at Tree House, I discovered another powerful tool for addressing childhood trauma. Mary described EMDR as "the best therapy there is for childhood of trauma, PTSD—oh, absolutely."

This resonated deeply with my own experience. Through my research and relationships with experts like Dr. Glenn Schiraldi (author of *The Adverse Childhood Experience Recovery Workbook*), I learned about the effectiveness of EMDR for processing traumatic memories. When my older brother Jamie revealed he had been suffering from depression for years despite seeing numerous doctors, Jamie finally sought EMDR therapy.

The results were remarkable. After just seven sessions with an EMDR specialist, Jamie's lifelong depression "shrunk to nothing." As I told Mary, "He's the happiest man now, and he wants to be the representative from UACT for EMDR, to promote it for childhood trauma."

This experience convinced me that specific, targeted interventions like EMDR can achieve in weeks what traditional talk therapy might take years to accomplish—if it succeeds at all. As Mary confirmed, "Talk therapy might work, but it takes forever. EMDR is almost automatic."

The Healing Power of Social Connection

A third crucial element of Tree House Recovery's approach addresses the social dimension of healing. They recognize that secure attachment and meaningful connection are not luxuries but biological necessities—particularly for those recovering from childhood trauma and addiction.

Justin spoke passionately about the importance of early attachment, suggesting that children who receive consistent, loving care during their first 18-24 months of life develop a neurobiological foundation that can buffer them against later adversity. He likened it to "the gorilla with the baby on the back," where the infant remains in close physical contact until they naturally begin to explore independence.

This perspective aligns with my own research into what I call "The Sacred 60"—the critical first 60 days of life during which the quality of attachment can profoundly influence a child's future resilience. As I've discovered, if a child receives loving care from a primary caregiver (usually the mother) during this crucial window, they develop neurological patterns that enable them to withstand significant adversity later in life.

Neal emphasized the importance of social connection: "Justin firmly believed isolation was probably one of the worst things that can happen. So the opposite of that was social connection, and we invented a bunch of tools in that realm."

For those who didn't receive this early foundation, Tree House Recovery creates a corrective experience through community. They foster deep social bonds among clients and staff, creating what attachment theorists would call a "secure base" from which individuals can explore emotional vulnerability and new ways of being.

When I asked Brent about the role of community in healing, he responded emphatically: "Even more important than [physical movement] is doing it with a group of like-minded people that understand you, and you understand them."

This sense of belonging and connection creates a context in which healing becomes possible. Brent described how the staff at Tree House model healthy relationships for clients: "I think it starts with us and the way that we interact with each other... they see that. I remember when I was a client, that was one thing that I really looked up to... seeing how they operated together... using that as role modeling, and it helped me aspire to be like that."

A particularly powerful aspect of this community is the open expression of love. When I asked Brent if they openly tell each other that they love each other, he responded: "Oh yeah. I do it all the time." This culture of expressed love extends to the clients as well, creating a healing environment where vulnerability and authentic connection can flourish.

The Healed Becoming the Healer

One of the most striking patterns that emerged from my conversations with Tree House staff is what Justin described as "the healed who becomes the healer." Brent's story exemplifies this journey: after graduating from the Tree House program, he was hired as a fitness coach, eventually working his way up to opening and directing a new Tree House location in his hometown of Wilmington, North Carolina.

Justin reflected on this phenomenon in correspondence after our initial conversations: "The healed who becomes the healer... I have been thinking of this a lot... Maybe the last step in healing for all of us is to take our own hardships and turn them into healing and growth for others. Pain into love."

This transformation from recipient to provider of healing reflects a profound truth about recovery: that finding purpose in helping others can itself be a powerful form of healing. As Brent explained: "We know what it's like to crawl out of darkness and build something first for ourselves, and we're basically reaching into other people's darkness and trying to pull them out of it, too."

This pattern echoes an ancient wisdom captured in various traditions. As the philosopher Friedrich Nietzsche expressed it: "He whose soul is deep through suffering, knowledge and power will find that the branches of his tree reach toward heaven only if its roots descend to hell." Our deepest wounds, when healed, can become our greatest sources of strength and wisdom.

Brent noted that this is a distinctive feature of the Tree House approach: "I think one of the things that makes our program special is the fact that a large percentage, I would say at least 90% of the people that work for Tree House are also in recovery. Have been through the program and understand it firsthand."

This creates a powerful authenticity in their work. As Justin observed: "It's the idea of the healed who becomes the healer... a legacy of stepping up in the face of hardship—not just for oneself, but for others—and finding purpose in alleviating suffering."

Addressing Childhood Trauma on a Larger Scale

When I asked Brent how we might collectively package and leverage healing and recovery to reach millions instead of thousands, his response was thought-provoking: "I think that would help, but I think that we would have to fundamentally change the entire way that this country is structured."

He pointed to cultural differences he observed during his travels: "If you go to a third world country, like Indonesia... they don't have the same kind of luxuries that we have. They're not as materialistic focused, they're not as independent, they're much more family oriented... they keep their families together, and they stay together. The way their towns are structured, they have elders, and it's just a completely different kind of structure than the way that we have it set up here."

Brent made a striking connection between America's founding ethos and the psychology of addiction: "Think of how this country was created. It was created based on settlers that came from different continents, coming here to discover, to seek, to start something new. And those principles, I think alone, are also principles that describe someone who struggles with addiction, like it's never good enough. You're constantly seeking something. You constantly want more and more and more."

This insight resonates with what a sociologist told me when I asked how we got here and how we solve the problem: "Our materialistic world is what has caused the trauma and addiction." As Brent observed, advanced civilization "has evolved based on advanced civilization, which sounds like it's made things worse, not better. Yes, we made things more convenient. But what it's done is it's disrupted a 10-million-year cycle of ancestral behavior" characterized by community, structure, accountability, and mutual support.

The Starfish Principle

When I asked George how Tree House Recovery addresses the stark reality that they can only serve a tiny fraction of those suffering from addiction, he shared the "starfish story" with me:

An elderly gentleman walking along the ocean's edge noticed a young boy bending down, picking up starfish, and throwing them back into the water. When asked what he was doing, the boy explained that he was saving the starfish from dying during low tide. The old man observed, "There must be thousands of them. You can't save them all." As the boy pitched another starfish into the ocean, he replied simply, "I just saved that one!"

This story captures the spirit of Tree House Recovery's approach to a seemingly insurmountable challenge. While they cannot single-handedly solve the epidemic of addiction, they can create transformative change for everyone they treat. And by developing and sharing their model through research and training, they extend their impact far beyond their direct services.

For those of us concerned with the broader crisis of childhood trauma, this principle offers both inspiration and guidance. We may not be able to immediately prevent all childhood trauma or heal all who suffer from its effects, but we can make meaningful differences in individual lives while working toward systemic change.

Implications for Addressing Childhood Trauma

Tree House Recovery's approach offers several important insights for our broader mission of addressing childhood trauma:

1. **Recognize Biological Diversity**: Just as individuals have different genetic predispositions to addiction, they may have varied neurobiological sensitivity to trauma. This perspective helps us move beyond one-size-fits-all approaches to both prevention and healing.

2. **Address Multiple Dimensions**: Effective interventions must consider biological, psychological, social, and spiritual factors simultaneously. Approaches that focus exclusively on one dimension may miss crucial opportunities for healing.

3. **Embrace Movement as Medicine**: As Dr. Ratey writes in "Spark," physical activity is not merely a healthy habit but "the single most powerful tool you have to optimize your brain function." Regular exercise produces changes in the brain's chemistry and structure that enhance learning, mood, and cognitive function—all critical components of trauma recovery.

4. **Create Structured Vulnerability**: Processes like Naked Writ-

ing offer safe, structured ways to approach painful material, allowing individuals to integrate traumatic experiences without becoming overwhelmed.

5. **Foster Deep Connection**: Secure attachment and meaningful relationships provide a neurobiological foundation for healing, helping to regulate stress responses and create safety for emotional processing.

6. **Utilize Targeted Interventions**: Approaches like EMDR can rapidly address traumatic memories that talk therapy alone might take years to process.

7. **Cultivate Gratitude**: Structured practices that foster gratitude may provide neurobiological benefits that counter the anhedonia often associated with trauma.

8. **Gather Data While Maintaining Heart**: Tree House Recovery's evolution shows how intuitive approaches can be refined through systematic data gathering without losing their humanistic core.

9. **Accept the Starfish Principle**: While addressing childhood trauma at a societal level remains our goal, we must also value the profound impact we can have on individual lives right now.

10. **Transform Pain into Purpose**: The pattern of the healed becoming healers suggests that finding meaning in our suffering by helping others may be an essential component of complete recovery.

Tree House Recovery reminds us that healing from childhood trauma is possible—not despite our biological makeup but through working with it intelligently. By understanding the complex interplay between genetics, environment, and personal psychology, we can develop approaches that transform vulnerability into strength and suffering into growth.

Their success in treating addiction—often considered one of the most challenging consequences of childhood trauma—offers hope that even deeply entrenched patterns can be changed with the right combination of understanding, support, and structured intervention. As we work toward a world where childhood trauma becomes increasingly rare, we can take inspiration from models like Tree House Recovery that show us how to heal what has already occurred.

In the words of Justin McMillen: "If you don't learn how to be you, you very easily could end up falling into addiction... The other answer could be to understand ourselves enough to know how to be ourselves within modernity, and understand that we're not built the same, and that for us, the rule book's different."

This insight applies not just to addiction but to all the varied manifestations of childhood trauma. By understanding our unique neurobiological makeup and learning to work with rather than against it, we can transform even the most painful experiences into pathways for growth and healing—or as Justin beautifully phrased it, turning "pain into love."

The suffering you endure because of childhood trauma does not have to be a life sentence. Recovery is not merely a possibility; it is a journey many have embarked upon and found success.

Amidst the early stages of developing effective healing interventions for the mental and biological consequences of trauma, I am filled with hope—a hope grounded in the promise of healing. I hope you feel empowered to seek help, support, or guidance for yourself or someone who may be silently suffering.

Together, we can break the cycle of trauma.

CHAPTER TWENTY-TWO

The Paradox of Childhood Trauma

Fuel for Resilience or a Path to Despair?

"I believe not only that trauma is curable, but that the healing process can be a catalyst for profound awakening."

–Peter A. Levine, PhD

WHILE WRITING MY MEMOIR, *The Kite That Couldn't Fly,* a burning question consumed me: Why did some of my siblings stumble under the weight of our childhood trauma yet succeed, while other siblings fell, and some were even crushed by the trauma?

Childhood trauma is a complex and multifaceted phenomenon that can have lasting implications on an individual's psyche and life trajectory. It is often depicted as a dark cloak that envelops a person from a young age, leading to feelings of shame, loneliness, and despair. Yet, paradoxically, there are those who manage to emerge from the depths of trauma, using the very experiences that sought to undermine them as fuel for extraordinary resilience and success. In exploring this paradox, we confront an essential question:

Why do some individuals flourish in the wake of such pain, while others remain mired in their suffering?

In her book, *The Unexpected Gift of Trauma*, author Dr. Edith Shiro examines the dynamics within this paradox, offering a compelling perspective on how trauma can oscillate between being both a catalyst for personal transformation and a debilitating burden. This discourse highlights the dual nature of trauma, essentially framing it as a double-edged sword, where the outcomes often hinge on a variety of factors including individual resilience, social support systems, coping mechanisms, and opportunities for healing.

We know precious little about why, but for some, trauma can act as a catalyst for exceptional success, functioning as a form of "jet fuel" that propels them toward achievement. This phenomenon can be seen in numerous high-profile figures who credit their challenging childhoods as fundamental to their drive, creativity, and perseverance. The emotional strife associated with trauma often instills a sense of urgency and determination that may not be present in those who have experienced more stable upbringings. The sheer will to overcome adversity can lead to remarkable accomplishments, transforming pain into passion, and suffering into strength.

As I reflect on this aspect of the paradox, I can draw from personal experiences and observations that reinforce this perspective. Many individuals, including myself, have utilized the emotional turbulence of childhood trauma to carve out paths that defy expectations. The fear of repeating the mistakes of the past or the longing for belonging and security can instill an acute desire to establish one's own identity or to succeed in realms previously deemed unattainable. In this regard, trauma becomes not only a source of pain but also a powerful motivator that can lead individuals to pursue their passions with unwavering tenacity.

However, it is crucial to recognize that the relationship between trauma and success is not linear. For many, as you have read throughout this book, the heavy toll of trauma can lead to psychological struggles that inhibit growth and development. Without the right resources, support, and opportunities for healing, the effects of childhood trauma can stifle potential and foster feelings of hopelessness and defeat. Some survivors find themselves caught in cycles of self-destructive behavior, failed relationships, and mental health challenges that leave them feeling prisoners of their past experiences.

The disparity in these trajectories illustrates a sobering reality: while some individuals may rise triumphantly from the ashes of trauma, others may become trapped within the emotional wreckage, unable to find a way out. Unfortunately, I can't find any data on who succeeds or struggles because of childhood trauma. I believe that those who thrive are likely a small minority.

In *The Unexpected Gift of Trauma*, Dr. Edith Shiro emphasizes the critical importance of support systems in determining which path an individual takes following traumatic experiences. Access to therapeutic resources, loving relationships, and nurturing environments can provide the scaffolding needed to transform trauma into a tool for growth. Conversely, a lack of these elements can exacerbate feelings of isolation and despair, making it even more difficult to escape the grip of trauma. This dichotomy highlights the notion that it is not the trauma itself that dictates an individual's outcome, but rather how one learns to navigate the complexities of healing in its wake.

Perhaps the most pertinent reflection on this paradox is the idea of agency. Those who harness their trauma as fuel for success often exhibit a profound sense of agency, demonstrating the ability to rewrite their narratives. They embrace their stories, channeling pain into art, activism, or entrepreneurial pursuits that not only propel them forward but inspire others as well. This transformation can illuminate paths of hope for many who have felt the shadow of trauma looming over their lives.

With the juxtaposed teaching principles of Mom and Dad, something almost magical happened. Dad did and said things that can only be explained as wrong, but some brilliance was mixed in with that wrong. I don't believe it was part of their parenting plan, but what played out in our lives might be explained by Carl Jung's belief: "No tree, it is said, can grow to heaven unless its roots reach down to hell."

Jung was not discussing hell, and he was not talking about heaven. Instead, he made an analogy of light opposing darkness, that every high must have a corresponding low. Maybe we needed the bad and tough lessons as something to push against to reach up.

It's a fact that storms and wind are required for the roots of a tree to grow bigger and stronger. If you prevent a tree from being moved by the wind, the roots won't grow as strong or deep, increasing the probability of the tree toppling and preventing the tree from reaching its ultimate height. Adversity is necessary for the tree to strengthen, allowing it to withstand even more harsh conditions. Did the adversity in our lives make us stronger?

Would I have been better off if I could remove all the bad from my childhood? Perhaps. But I fear all the happiness would be wiped out if I did. I'm proud of all my life experiences and will forever hold my uniqueness high in the air, just as I held the trophy I won with the kite that couldn't fly.

The Sacred 60: Maybe A Key to the Trauma Paradox

The question that haunted me throughout writing *The Kite That Couldn't Fly* continues to echo: why did some of my siblings and I rise above our shared childhood trauma while others crumbled beneath its weight? This paradox—where identical adversity produces dramatically different outcomes—may find partial explanation in what neuroscience has recently revealed about our earliest days of life.

Those first 60 days after birth—what I've come to call "The Sacred 60"—appear to create a neurobiological foundation that influences how we respond to future adversity. During this critical window, the infant brain is rapidly forming connections that will shape stress response patterns for decades to come. When a baby receives consistent, loving care during this period, their developing nervous system learns that the world, despite its challenges, is fundamentally safe.

Reflecting on my family's story through this lens offers a compelling possibility. As the second born in our family of 14, I benefited from my mother's relatively undivided attention during those crucial early weeks. Jamie, as the firstborn, likely received similar focused nurturing. Our mother's warm gaze, gentle touch, and responsive care during those first 60 days may have gifted us with an invisible armor—a neurological resilience that would later help us withstand the storms of our difficult childhood.

But what of Patrick and Adam, my brothers who eventually lost their battles with addiction? Born later in the birth order, they arrived into a home already stretched thin by the demands of caring for so many children. Our loving mother, despite her best intentions, simply couldn't provide the same quality of one-on-one attention during their critical developmental window. By then, her energy was divided among many children, her stress levels undoubtedly higher, and her capacity for the kind of sustained, attuned interaction that builds secure attachment necessarily diminished.

This isn't about assigning blame—our mother loved all her children profoundly. Rather, it's about understanding how biological factors might intersect with lived experience to create different outcomes from shared circumstances. Without that early neurological "vaccination" against adversity, Patrick and Adam may have been more vulnerable to the trauma that would later envelop our household.

Dr. Bruce Perry's research supports this theory, showing that emotional neglect in those first 60 days—even when unintentional and caused by circumstances beyond a parent's control—can leave children particularly susceptible to the effects of later trauma.[10] Their stress response systems never develop the regulation patterns that might have protected them, making it harder to bounce back from adversity.

This insight doesn't provide a complete explanation for why some trauma survivors thrive while others struggle—many factors including genetics, temperament, timing of trauma, and access to healing resources all play roles. But it does offer a compelling piece of the puzzle that aligns with both scientific research and my family's lived experience.

The paths my siblings and I took weren't simply matters of willpower or character. They may have been influenced by neurobiological foundations laid before any of us had formed conscious memories—during those sacred 60 days when our brains were learning their first and most powerful lessons about the world.

This perspective doesn't diminish the tragedy of losing Patrick and Adam. If anything, it deepens my compassion for their struggles and strengthens my resolve to help others understand the profound importance of early attachment. It also highlights why supporting new parents and infants must be a cornerstone of any serious effort to prevent childhood trauma and its devastating aftereffects.

Perhaps in this understanding lies not just an explanation for the past, but a powerful direction for the future—a way to ensure more children develop the neurological resilience that turns adversity into strength rather than destruction.

Do not misunderstand me—I do not suggest there is any benefit to being exposed to childhood trauma, it should never be a selected path to success. While trauma can catapult some to success, that does not always mean those people do not require or would not benefit from healing therapies.

The paradox of childhood trauma presents a compelling examination of human resilience and vulnerability. Trauma can serve as both a hindrance and an empowering force, dictating divergent paths for those it touches. *The Unexpected Gift of Trauma* captures this complexity, shining a light on the intricate interplay between suffering and success. While it acknowledges the difficulty of the journey, it also celebrates the incredible capacity for transformation that lies within us all.

As we navigate our own experiences with trauma, let us recognize and embrace the duality of our struggles. They may ultimately lead us to discover not just survival, but the extraordinary power of thriving in the face of adversity.

Book III
A Proclamation for Change

As we reach the concluding section of *Greater Than Gravity: How Childhood Trauma is Pulling Down Humanity*, I invite you to pause and reflect on the insights and revelations we've explored throughout the first two books.

In Book I, we meticulously documented the multifaceted nature of childhood trauma—what it is, the destruction it perpetuates, and the alarming prevalence of this issue not only in the United States but globally. We uncovered the untold stories and statistics that paint a troubling picture of how trauma shapes lives and societies.

In Book II, we transitioned into an examination of healing—what has fallen short in addressing the needs of those affected by trauma and what has been effective. Drawing from my personal experiences and research, I provided a comprehensive understanding of the therapeutic approaches available, as well as the systemic barriers that often hinder recovery. In these chapters, I endeavored to take on the role of a reporter, diligently presenting the facts and findings, even as the emotional weight of the subject matter frequently pulled me back into my own story. I believe it is crucial to base our understanding of healing from trauma on a solid foundation of evidence and shared experiences.

In Book III, we pivot from understanding to action, transforming knowledge into a powerful manifesto for change. Moving beyond observation and healing strategies, I step into the role of advocate and activist to call for a unified, global effort to end childhood trauma. This final section presents a transformative vision where childhood trauma becomes a relic of the past.

While concrete plans will emerge, with the help of experts and leaders, we first must embrace the boundless possibilities that lie ahead. Together, we can forge new pathways toward safe, nurturing environments for future generations. This vision is not just an aspiration, but an achievable reality.

This is our collective awakening to what can be. Join me on a journey that demands the participation of every individual committed to transforming how we protect and nurture our children.

CHAPTER TWENTY-THREE

Creating the "Tipping Point"

"A change of worldview can change the world viewed."

–Joseph Chilton Pearce

IN THE REALM OF visionary aspirations, the phrase "Big Hairy Audacious Goal" was brought to life by Jim Collins and Jerry Porras in their groundbreaking book, *Built to Last: Successful Habits of Visionary Companies*. In their book, the authors illustrated the necessity of setting daring goals to forge a powerful vision and sustain a competitive edge. This concept has since permeated the worlds of business and personal development, encouraging individuals and organizations alike to stretch beyond the conventional and strive for the extraordinary.

A "Big Hairy Audacious Goal" (BHAG) is not merely a target; it is a stake in the ground for inspiration and motivation. It represents a bold challenge—a compelling vision that demands brilliance, innovation, and a commitment to push boundaries. A true BHAG captivates the imagination to such an extent that it necessitates monumental leaps in thought and action.

After penning the first two books of this journey, I found myself besieged by a haunting question:

What now?

I'm hopeful this question resonates with you as well.

The weight of a profound responsibility that now rests upon our shoulders. As Elie Wiesel poignantly stated, "We are each responsible for the evil we do not prevent." Wiesel, a Holocaust survivor and tireless advocate for human rights, imparted a crucial truth: inaction in the presence of injustice is complicity in its perpetuation.

Together, we have determined that we are living amid an epidemic of childhood trauma, and we must hit the panic button. We must now confront the pressing question: What do we do next?

It is time for us to rise to the occasion and craft a revolutionary vision for our society. United Against Childhood Trauma (UACT) is the rallying cry for our movement, and our Big Hairy Audacious Goal is crystal clear: ending childhood trauma. Let us join forces and ignite the change our world desperately needs.

The time for action is now.

Ending childhood trauma must be our unwavering goal. I can almost hear the skepticism in the air.

"Are you crazy?"

I assure you; I am not. I understand how grandiose and incredibly challenging this aim is. It may even seem impossibly lofty. Yet, that's exactly where the power lies.

BHAGs hold a unique magic. They inspire us to expand our minds and push the boundaries of what we believe is possible. When we set our sights on these monumental aspirations, we don't just chase a distant target; we embark on a transformative journey that can alter the very fabric of our lives and communities.

Tony Robbins makes a compelling case for the pursuit of seemingly unreal goals. He emphasizes that the true value lies not in the attainment of the BHAG itself, but in the profound personal growth that occurs along the way. The process of striving toward these ambitious objectives shifts our mindset, molds our character, and ignites passions we may have never known existed within us.

This requires a cultivation of resilience, creativity, and a fierce determination that will ripple out into our communities. Each step we take, no matter how small, sends out shockwaves of change, inspiring others to join in the fight against childhood trauma. The journey elevates not just ourselves, but also those around us, creating a movement that will reverberate through generations.

So, yes, I admit this is an impossible goal. Yet in aiming for it, I ask you to commit to a shared vision that can mobilize countless hearts and minds. Let's harness the magic of this audacious goal to create and fuel our mission, challenge the status quo, and drive real change. Together, we have the power to redefine the narrative around childhood trauma and create a brighter, healthier future for the generations to come. It's time to embrace this journey—unwavering and united—in our quest to end childhood trauma.

In the spirit of Malcolm Gladwell's concept of *The Tipping Point*, we find ourselves on the brink of a revolution against childhood trauma—a movement poised to transform society in profound ways. The tipping point is where the unexpected becomes the expected, and radical change shifts from a mere dream to an undeniable certainty.

Imagine a diverse community of passionate individuals, united by a Big Hairy Audacious Goal to eradicate childhood trauma once and for all. This collective purpose serves as the catalyst for change, energizing each participant to push boundaries and challenge conventional thinking. As we rally together with this vision, we create a powerful momentum that cannot be ignored.

The synergy among us will act as the spark needed to ignite a broader movement. Each action we take—whether it be raising awareness, advocating for policy reform, or supporting trauma-informed practices in our communities—contributes to a ripple effect. As these ripples converge, they create the critical mass required to reach that tipping point in which change becomes inevitable.

As we persevere toward our BHAG, we will establish new norms, alter public perception, and inspire others to join us in this mission. The momentum will dismantle the entrenched systems that perpetuate trauma and cultivate an environment where healing and resilience prevail.

So let us embrace the transformative power of our collective vision. Together, we can reach the tipping point where the dream of ending childhood trauma becomes a tangible reality, and a new era of hope and healing is born. In this world, our audacious goal will no longer seem radical; it will become the foundation for the brighter future we all desire.

Lessons from History: Learning from Our Public Health Victories

All meaningful change begins with awareness, for it is only when we shine a light on the silent suffering of childhood trauma that we can galvanize the understanding and support necessary to transform our society into a nurturing environment for every child, and every adult.

Throughout history, the US has faced numerous public health crises, and time and again, we have risen to the challenge, demonstrating that with focus, collaboration, and determination, we can turn the tide against even the most daunting health threats. As I reflect on the transformative triumphs of our nation's public health interventions, I am struck by the immense power we hold when we unite to address societal health issues. This collective action has not only saved lives but has also instilled hope and resilience within our communities.

Take, for instance, the monumental efforts to combat smoking-related diseases that began in the 1960s. When Dr. Luther Terry, then the Surgeon General, released the landmark report on smoking and health, it served as a wake-up call that galvanized the nation. Smoking cessation became a priority, leading to warning labels on cigarette packs, advertising restrictions, and public smoking bans. Through tenacious campaigns like "The Real Cost" and "Tips From Former Smokers," we witnessed a seismic shift in public perception about tobacco.

The fruits of these efforts are undeniable: the adult smoking rate plummeted from approximately 42% in 1965 to around 14% in 2019, and an estimated 800,000 deaths from lung cancer were prevented during that time. This triumph exemplifies how concerted public health initiatives can lessen a health crisis when we leverage our collective willpower and resources. Was smoking eliminated? No. But just think of the millions who have avoided cancer and heart disease.

Similarly, the fight against polio showcased our nation's ability to mobilize for a greater purpose. The introduction of the polio vaccine in the 1950s marked a pivotal moment in public health history. Mass immunization campaigns saw the incidence of polio decrease from over 20,000 cases annually to virtually zero by the 1970s, culminating in the declaration of polio's eradication in the US in 1979. Witnessing a disease that once paralyzed thousands evaporate from our society was a testament to our capability for positive change when we align our focus toward common goals.

The response to the HIV epidemic provides another powerful example of public health resilience. Beginning in the 1980s, we faced a crisis that threatened to disrupt lives and communities across the nation. Yet, through education, safe sex campaigns, and the introduction of antiretroviral therapy, we transformed the narrative surrounding HIV. The dramatic 73% decrease in new HIV diagnoses from 1984 to 2019 illustrates what is possible when we embrace innovation and collaborative action in public health.

However, despite these inspirational feats of public health, it is disheartening to find that a similar commitment has yet to materialize in the fight against childhood trauma—a pervasive and persistent public health crisis that is orders of magnitude greater than smoking, polio and HIV combined, that remains largely unaddressed. The groundbreaking Adverse Childhood Experiences (ACEs) study, published in the late 1990s, illuminated the deep and lasting consequences of childhood trauma. Twenty-six years later, our coordinated efforts to prevent child abuse at systemic levels have been almost nonexistent. Millions of children continue to suffer from abuse each year, and the scars of trauma, often invisible, afflict an estimated 180 million adults in the US alone.

The lack of progress can be attributed to various factors: underfunded social support systems, insufficient training for professionals working with at-risk families, and a dearth of comprehensive public awareness campaigns. Without structured policy frameworks and measurable goals, our attempts to address the issue remain fragmented and ineffective. The time has come for us to confront this painful reality with urgency and determination.

In the pursuit of eradicating childhood trauma, it is imperative that we elevate this cause to a national priority. We must galvanize a collective and coordinated strategy that mirrors the successful public health interventions we have seen in the past. This initiative demands not only our attention but actionable steps that bring together policymakers, health professionals, educators, and communities to forge a united front against this crisis.

My mission is clear: Raise awareness about the profound impact of childhood trauma and to advocate for collective action that creates effective solutions. I hope to foster understanding and compassion in our society, compelling us to build nurturing environments for all children. We have the power to break the cycle of trauma, transforming pain into resilience and suffering into strength.

It's time to turn up the volume on this critical issue and place it before the eyes of the nation. With an unwavering commitment to our children's well-being, we can mobilize resources and leadership, create a comprehensive national plan, and redefine our approach to childhood trauma. History has shown us that when America focuses on solving societal health issues, remarkable progress can be made. Together, we have the power to change the narrative and ensure that every child has the chance to thrive.

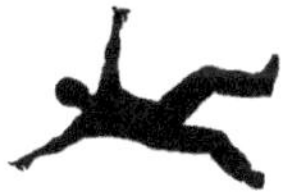

Dr. Lee Long is a friend, colleague, founder and CEO of Restoration Counseling. Lee is a pioneer in the field of recovery from childhood trauma, possessing a remarkable ability to convey complex concepts through metaphors and stories. In one of my first meetings with Dr. Lee, he employed a powerful analogy of a polluted river to illustrate what it will take to end childhood trauma.

Imagine a vibrant community nestled alongside a flowing river, its banks teeming with life. However, this river, once a source of nourishment and joy, has become tragically polluted. The residents, unaware of the contamination, go about their daily lives, using the river's water for drinking, cooking, and washing. The children, full of innocence and trust, drink deeply from its depths, blissfully unaware of the danger that lurks within.

As time passes, the effects of the pollution begin to manifest. The children who have ingested the tainted water become sick, their vitality sapped by an illness that, if left untreated, will shadow them for the rest of their lives. This sickness represents the long-term emotional and psychological repercussions of childhood trauma. Just as the pollutants in the river threaten the health of the community, unaddressed childhood trauma endangers the well-being of the children and future generations.

Recognizing the crisis, the elders of the community gather to seek a solution. Their first step is to raise awareness: they inform the villagers about the invisible threat of the polluted water and the illness it causes. It is a difficult conversation, for admitting that the very source of life has become a harbinger of sickness requires vulnerability and courage. Awareness becomes the beacon of hope; it is the first step toward communal healing. Only when the community acknowledges the problem can they begin to act.

Next, the elders focus on treating those who are already suffering from the effects of the contaminated water. They establish a treatment center along the riverbank where trained healers provide care and support to the sick children, offering remedies to alleviate their symptoms and assist in their recovery. This act of treating the ill embodies the commitment to healing, acknowledging the wounds inflicted by trauma and providing a pathway for restoration.

Yet, the elders know that while raising awareness and treating the sick are crucial, true change requires a more profound solution. They must go upstream—journalists, educators, and environmental advocates unite to identify and eliminate the sources of pollution that are entering the river. They work diligently to understand how the pollutants originated, instituting stricter regulations to prevent further contamination. This effort represents the prevention of future trauma, safeguarding the health of the entire community and ensuring that the next generation can thrive free from the shadows of their predecessors' experiences.

In the end, the actions of the elders draw a clear connection between awareness, healing, and prevention—the three key tenets required to eradicate childhood trauma. Raising awareness about the reality of trauma is paramount; acknowledging its effects invites healing not only for the individual but for the entire community. Through interventional treatment, we can address the pain inflicted by past experiences, empowering those affected to reclaim their lives. Finally, by preventing further trauma, we protect future generations from suffering the same fate.

Just as the river gains purity and strength through the collective efforts of the elders and the community, so too can we create an environment in which children are nurtured, supported, and free to flourish. Ending childhood trauma is not just a matter of addressing the past; it involves a commitment to a brighter future for all through awareness, healing, and prevention.

CHAPTER TWENTY-FOUR

Awareness

The First Step Toward Ending Childhood Trauma

"Making an injury visible and public is often the first step in remedying it, and political change often follows culture, as what was tolerated is seen to be intolerable, or what was overlooked becomes obvious."

–Rebecca Solnit, Hope in the Dark

AWARENESS IS THE CORNERSTONE of change; it is the catalyst that ignites the transformation of societies, individuals, and systems. Just as a seed must first be recognized for its potential before it can blossom into a flower, we must first acknowledge the reality of childhood trauma to pave the way for healing and resilience. The journey toward ending childhood trauma begins with awareness—a conscious recognition of its prevalence, consequences, and the urgent need for action.

Let's explore how awareness can become the driving force behind collective efforts to address and ultimately eradicate childhood trauma.

Understanding the Scale of Childhood Trauma

Before we can effectively tackle childhood trauma, we must first understand its magnitude. We've learned how billions of children worldwide experience various forms of trauma, from emotional and physical abuse to neglect and other adverse childhood experiences (ACEs). By raising awareness about the scope and impact of these experiences, we equip communities with the knowledge needed to identify warning signs and intervene early. When individuals recognize the signs of trauma, they become empowered to act. That can look like offering support to affected children, advocating for policy change, or simply fostering conversations about mental health within their circles.

Educating the Public & Professionals

Awareness is not solely about acknowledging trauma; it also involves educating ourselves and others. This education must target not only the public but also professionals who interact with children—educators, healthcare providers, social workers, and community leaders. Equipping these individuals with the knowledge and skills to recognize trauma can help create supportive environments for children and families. Training programs that emphasize trauma-informed practices are essential to ensure that everyone from teachers to therapists can respond appropriately and compassionately. By fostering a culture of understanding, we can build a community that is responsive to the needs of children and addresses trauma with empathy and expertise.

Promoting Conversations Around Trauma

Creating an awareness of childhood trauma also means encouraging open conversations. The stigma surrounding trauma can often silence sufferers and prevent them from seeking help. We must challenge these taboos and foster environments where individuals feel safe to share their experiences. Through storytelling, community forums, and awareness campaigns, we can amplify voices that have long been unheard. These dialogues not only validate the experiences of those affected but also educate others on the lasting impacts of trauma. By building a culture of openness, we create spaces where healing can occur, and prevention can flourish. I hope this book has armed you and has provided the impetus and the courage to have such conversations.

The Interconnectedness of Awareness, Healing, & Prevention

It's crucial to recognize the overlapping nature of awareness, healing, and prevention in the fight to end childhood trauma. Awareness is the bridge that connects these pillars. Without awareness, treatment efforts may be misdirected or ineffective, as individuals may not recognize the signs of trauma or its underlying causes. Similarly, preventive measures rely on awareness to inform communities of risk factors and protective strategies. Education and outreach initiatives can illuminate the ways in which trauma can manifest and encourage proactive steps to mitigate its effects. Increasing awareness not only contributes directly to treatment strategies but also enhances prevention efforts.

When communities come together to cultivate awareness, they create a ripple effect that enhances the efficacy of treatment and strengthens preventive measures. Education empowers families to take an active role in supporting their children and seeking help when needed. Moreover, when people know how to identify trauma, they can advocate more effectively for systemic changes that support child welfare in schools, hospitals, and communities.

Let's dream and brainstorm for a moment. What could we do to accelerate awareness to the childhood trauma pandemic we face? Let's assume we have unlimited resources to drive massive, transformational awareness about childhood trauma. Here are the top five ideal communication vehicles we could utilize:

1. **Documentary Film Series:** Create a powerful documentary series showcasing real-life stories of individuals affected by childhood trauma. Additionally, include experts discussing the psychological, emotional, and societal implications of these experiences. Leverage platforms like Netflix and Hulu to reach a wide audience, making the series accessible globally and sparking conversations.

2. **Social Media Campaigns:** Launch a comprehensive social media campaign across multiple platforms (Instagram, Facebook, TikTok, X, LinkedIn, and relevant others) focusing on educational content, survivor stories, expert interviews, and interactive resources. Collaborate with influencers, mental health advocates, and organizations to amplify messages, create viral challenges, and host live events that encourage community engagement and sharing.

3. **National Awareness Events:** Organize large-scale events, such as a national conference or festival dedicated to childhood trauma awareness, featuring keynote speakers, workshops, panel discussions, and artistic expressions (e.g., performances, art exhibits) that convey personal stories and expert insights. This would not only create awareness but also foster community connection and collaboration among

stakeholders. Imagine National UACT Day where every sufferer and survivor wore the UACT tee shirt, and the proceeds of the tee shirts help fund the movement.

4. **Virtual Reality (VR) Experiences:** Develop immersive VR experiences that allow users to walk in the shoes of individuals who have experienced childhood trauma. This innovative approach can evoke empathy and understanding in a profound way, making the effects of trauma more tangible. These experiences could be featured in schools, community centers, and public spaces to reach diverse audiences.

5. **Comprehensive Educational Programs:** Fund and implement educational programs in schools, workplaces, and community organizations focusing on trauma awareness, mental health literacy, and resilience-building. These programs could include workshops, curriculum development, and resources for both children and adults to ensure broad-based understanding and proactive approaches to prevention and treatment. Just imagine an AI-enabled application that spoke to the participant in their language offering escalating interactive training modules based on the participants' needs.

Currently, there is a lack of available data on the level of awareness surrounding childhood trauma. My limited observations suggest that as a nation, our understanding of this issue is minimal. I can illustrate this with my own experience: despite growing up amid complex childhood trauma, I didn't become aware of it until I was 70 years old. Based on this, I estimate that the current awareness of childhood trauma and adverse childhood experiences (ACEs) is likely below 5%.

Fast forward. Imagine we are setting a goal of having 50% of Americans commonly understand what childhood trauma is by 2030, 75% by 2035, and 95% by 2050.

I am confident that by fostering effective awareness around childhood trauma, we can ignite a meaningful conversation that inspires individuals and communities to actively engage in both treatment and prevention efforts. To achieve this ambitious vision, we can utilize targeted communication vehicles to create a comprehensive approach. By driving awareness, fostering understanding, and encouraging action, we can significantly combat childhood trauma on a large scale.

Chapter Twenty-Five
An Ounce of Prevention...

"An ounce of prevention is worth a pound of cure."

–Benjamin Franklin

THE PHRASE "AN OUNCE of prevention is worth a pound of cure" is most famously associated with Benjamin Franklin's writings on the importance of preventive measures, particularly in healthcare and public health. This quotation succinctly encapsulates the idea that taking proactive steps to prevent a problem is far more effective—and less burdensome—than trying to fix it after it has occurred.

Childhood trauma is a pervasive issue that affects hundreds of millions of children worldwide, leaving lasting scars that can influence their mental health, social development, and overall well-being. While awareness and healing strategies are crucial components in the journey of recovery as covered in the previous two chapters, prevention stands out as the most potent means of curbing the prevalence of childhood trauma. By establishing robust frameworks and interventions that prevent trauma before it occurs, society can foster healthier environments for children, enabling them to thrive, free from the debilitating impacts of adverse experiences.

Prevention is the second pillar in addressing childhood trauma. In this chapter, we'll discuss innovative approaches to create effective prevention strategies.

The Case for Prevention

Preventing childhood trauma is essential not only for the well-being of individual children but also for the long-term health of communities and society as a whole. As you have discovered in the previous chapters, childhood trauma can lead to a myriad of negative outcomes, including mental health disorders, substance abuse, and even increased risk for criminal behavior. The economic implications are also staggering, as the costs associated with treating trauma-related issues can far exceed the investment required for preventive measures. Furthermore, societal attitudes toward prevention can set the foundation for a cultural shift that normalizes support for children and families facing high-risk situations.

Let's let our minds wonder about possible strategies for prevention.

1. The First 60 Days of Life:

For parents, who they are is more important than what they are doing.

In their book, *Trauma Through a Child's Eyes*, authors Levine and Kline make the compelling point that when it comes to preventing childhood trauma the parent's first responsibly is to attend to her or his own emotional state, since it's only the adult's calm, competent, and reassuring presence that children find the space to resolved their tensions.

The implications are clear: society must protect and support the mother-infant bond during this crucial period.

Dr. Gordon Neufeld is a developmental psychologist and founder of the Neufeld Institute and has spent decades studying child development, attachment theory, and the conditions needed for healthy emotional growth. Neufeld believes human potential unfolds spontaneously but isn't inevitable. Creating the conditions for healthy emotional development isn't just about preventing trauma—it's about building the capacity to handle future challenges with resilience.[117]

These findings demand we move beyond viewing early nurturing as simply desirable to recognizing it as biologically essential. When we understand that a baby's nervous system expects and requires consistent loving care to develop properly, we see that meeting these needs isn't optional—it's as fundamental as providing food or shelter.

The science is unequivocal: those first 60 days set a trajectory that shapes all future development. While later experiences matter, nothing can fully replace the foundation built through early, consistent maternal nurturing. This understanding must guide how we support new mothers and protect the sacred space of early bonding.

2. Supportive Family & Parenting Programs:

Implementing family-centered programs that provide support and resources can significantly reduce the occurrence of traumatic experiences. These programs can include early parenting classes that teach effective communication and nurturing skills, family counseling services to help resolve conflict, and access to social support networks. By strengthening family units, children are more likely to experience stable and nurturing environments that mitigate the risk of trauma.

3. Community-based Initiatives:

Prevention efforts can be amplified through community engagement. Local governments and organizations should invest in community centers that offer recreational activities, mentorship programs, and safe spaces for children. Engaging the community fosters connections and support systems that provide children a sense of belonging, reducing their vulnerability to trauma. In *The Deepest Well*, Dr. Burke emphasizes how mindfulness practices can profoundly enhance overall well-being by promoting emotional resilience and reducing stress. She illustrates that incorporating mindfulness into daily life not only fosters a deeper connection to oneself but also cultivates healthier relationships and improved mental clarity, ultimately leading to a more fulfilled and purposeful life.

4. Mental Health Resources:

Enhancing the availability of mental health resources for families can preemptively address issues that may lead to trauma. Schools should have access to school-based mental health professionals who can work with children and their families to recognize early signs of distress and promote prevention. Early intervention services can provide essential coping strategies and emotional support, ultimately preventing situation escalation that could result in trauma.

5. Collaborative Policy Advocacy:

To create a sustainable impact, stakeholders must advocate for policies that prioritize child welfare and trauma prevention. This includes pushing for reforms in child protection laws, advocating for funding for social services, and supporting legislation that promotes mental health awareness. Collaboration between policymakers, educators, health professionals, and community organizations is necessary to create frameworks that protect at-risk children and families.

6. Trauma-Informed Care in Schools:

Schools play a critical role in preventing trauma among children. Implementing trauma-informed practices within educational settings ensures that staff are trained to recognize and respond to the signs of trauma effectively. Creating a school culture that emphasizes emotional safety, respect, and inclusivity can help mitigate the impacts of trauma on students.

7. Promoting Resilience:

Building resilience in children is a foundational aspect of trauma prevention. Programs focused on life skills training, emotional literacy, and problem-solving can empower children to handle adversities more effectively. Equipping children with these tools not only helps them cope with challenges but also fosters a sense of agency, thereby decreasing their susceptibility to trauma.

Preventing childhood trauma requires a sophisticated understanding of how early experiences shape human development. Prevention must begin with supporting caregivers themselves. Much of our work may well start in the home. This is because a parent's emotional state directly impacts their child's ability to process and resolve tension.

Our path forward demands a holistic approach that weaves together individual and family support, community engagement, and policy reform. This connects to broader initiatives like trauma-informed schools and mental health resources, creating a network of support that doesn't just prevent trauma but actively cultivates resilience.

The wisdom in prevention isn't just about avoiding harm—it's about creating the conditions where human potential can fully flourish, transforming the adage, "An ounce of prevention is worth a pound of cure," from a simple truism into a roadmap for societal transformation.

Chapter Twenty-Six

Raising the Bar

The Need for a Next-Generation ACEs Tool

"Good is the enemy of great."

–Jim Collins

In every facet of life, the pursuit of excellence demands a commitment to continuous improvement. When we uncover a tool or practice that proves beneficial, it's easy to become complacent, believing that we have reached a satisfactory endpoint. However, history has shown us that stagnation often occurs when we settle for good enough, allowing it to overshadow our potential for greatness.

The reality is that innovation and progress thrive on a foundation of constant evaluation and enhancement. When we recognize the value we generate through our offerings, it becomes imperative to seek out opportunities for refinement and evolution. To elevate our impact and maximize the benefits we provide, we must challenge ourselves to push beyond merely acceptable solutions and relentlessly aspire to greatness.

Embracing this mindset not only transforms our work but also inspires those around us to strive for a higher standard, igniting a ripple effect of improvement and achievement that extends far beyond our initial goals.

A Next-Generation ACEs Assessment Tool

By now you know the work of Drs. Felitti and Anda in the Adverse Childhood Experiences (ACEs) study revolutionized our understanding of the prevalence of and profound impact that childhood trauma can have on lifelong health and well-being. This groundbreaking work not only identified a connection between adverse childhood experiences and various negative health outcomes but also ignited a movement dedicated to understanding and addressing the roots of these experiences.

As practitioners, researchers, and advocates have sought to apply the knowledge gained from the ACEs study over the past three decades, it has become increasingly evident that while the original ACEs assessment tool was transformative, it is now in need of modernization to reflect current research, social dynamics, technological advances, and the evolving landscape of mental and metabolic health.

Despite the monumental value of the ACEs tool, numerous scholars, clinicians, and mental health professionals have identified limitations in its original framework, emphasizing the necessity for a next-generation version.

The primary criticism lies in the original tool's narrow focus on 10 specified adverse experiences, which, while significant, does not account for the broader spectrum of trauma and adversity that individuals may face in today's complex societal context. For instance, factors such as systemic racism, socio-economic disparities, and the impact of technology on childhood experiences were either overlooked or underrepresented in the original instrument. This limited scope risks failing to capture the nuanced realities of today's youth and undermines the tool's potential for comprehensive application in diverse populations.

Another critical area for improvement is the ACEs tool's lack of cultural sensitivity. The original survey was primarily developed within a specific demographic, which may not adequately reflect the experiences of marginalized communities. Researchers have argued that a modernized version of the ACEs assessment must prioritize inclusivity and cultural relevance by incorporating a broader array of experiences and tailoring questions to resonate with different sociocultural contexts. This adaptability would enhance the survey's utility as a universal tool for assessment and support across diverse populations.

In addition, the original ACEs assessment relies heavily on self-reported data, which can be subject to biases and inaccuracies. Individuals may underreport their experiences due to shame, stigma, or fear of judgment. An updated version of the ACEs tool could incorporate additional methodologies, such as qualitative interviews or observational assessments, to provide a more nuanced and accurate understanding of experiences of adversity.

Finally, I want to share an observation that I have yet to encounter in the existing literature, which leads me to believe that the current assessment tool does not provide a comprehensive understanding of adverse childhood experiences. The original ACEs assessment fails to capture the intensity and frequency of these experiences. For instance, question #3 of the original survey asks, "Did an adult or person at least five years older than you ever touch or fondle you or have you touch their body in a sexual way? Or attempt or actually have oral, anal, or vaginal intercourse with you?"

Consider respondent A, who experienced inappropriate touching once by an older neighbor boy. She would receive an ACE score of

1. Now, look at respondent B, who suffered repeated sexual assault by multiple family members. She too would receive a score of 1. While it may seem instinctual that respondent B endured a far more damaging trauma, the current tool does not account for this nuance, and both individuals end up with the same score and based on that score, receive the same treatment and or attention.

Imagine if, for each of the 10 domains (or whatever the new number may be), there were follow-up questions focusing on the frequency and intensity of these traumatic experiences. This enhancement could result in scores exceeding 10, allowing for greater differentiation among respondents and offering a more nuanced view of the impact of adverse experiences.

As we reflect on these limitations, the challenge now is not to critique the original ACEs survey, but to develop a version that harnesses the transformative potential of this pioneering work while addressing its shortcomings. Despite the clear need for modernization, no formal proposals have emerged for a next-generation ACEs tool that integrates the wealth of knowledge gained from decades of research. This gap presents a unique opportunity for collaboration among researchers, clinicians, and communities to co-create a more comprehensive and effective tool that reflects the intricate realities of contemporary childhood experiences.

The time has come for us to honor the legacy of Felitti and Anda by taking the next step in the evolution of the ACEs framework. By engaging in a rigorous process of research, dialogue, and community involvement, we can develop an enhanced ACEs assessment that not only honors the original intent of the tool but also expands its reach and applicability. Doing so would empower practitioners to better identify and support individuals facing adversity, fostering resilience and healing in a more responsive and relevant manner.

In a world that continually evolves, so too must our tools for understanding and addressing trauma. It is time for the next generation of the ACEs assessment tool to emerge, reflecting the complexities of modern childhood while providing a robust framework for intervention and support.

What You Measure Gets Better

"In God we trust; all others bring data."

–W. Edwards Deming

The adage "what you measure gets better" encapsulates a fundamental principle. If you seek to improve *anything*, you first need a baseline. While the origins of this phrase can be traced back to quality management practices in industries, notably popularized by management consultant Peter Drucker, its application extends far beyond business. In the context of childhood trauma, the saying highlights the critical need for comprehensive data collection and analysis to effectively understand, address, and ultimately reduce the impact of trauma on young lives.

The essence of "what you measure gets better" conveys a powerful idea: when we actively monitor our efforts, we can react to trends, recognize successes, and identify problems that require intervention. For instance, in healthcare, measuring patient outcomes leads to improved treatment protocols. In education, tracking student performance informs pedagogical strategies. This principle operates on the premise that measurement creates accountability and drives continuous improvement. It reminds us that to achieve tangible progress in any area, a systematic approach to gathering and interpreting data is essential.

The Case for Data in Addressing Childhood Trauma

When applied to the challenge of childhood trauma, this maxim becomes a call to deliberately enhance our understanding of the scope, causes, prevalence and effects of trauma on children. We know precious little about the prevalence and trends of childhood trauma.

Is it getting better or worse? We don't know. (Although some research suggests trauma prevalence is growing.)

Are our programs and improvement initiatives working? We don't know.

The necessity for data—specifically, the collection, management, data visualization and tracking of vast amounts of information—comes into sharp focus when we consider how we can use this information to inform our policies and interventions.

Comprehensive Assessment

Collecting extensive data about childhood trauma enables a deeper comprehension of its prevalence and causes. National surveys, community assessments, and research studies can quantify how many children are affected, what types of traumas they experience, and the demographics most at risk. By aggregating this information, stakeholders can develop a comprehensive picture of the problem, leading to targeted solutions.

Identifying Patterns & Trends

With regular data collection, we can identify patterns and trends over time regarding the incidence and impact of childhood trauma. By analyzing this data, patterns may emerge that reveal specific vulnerabilities within certain demographics, geographic areas, or social situations. Such insights help policymakers prioritize resources and tailor interventions where they are needed most.

Monitoring Program Effectiveness

Data plays a pivotal role in assessing the effectiveness of programs and interventions designed to prevent and alleviate childhood trauma. Frequent evaluation through data collection allows organizations to track progress, understand what strategies are working, and identify those that require modification. As programs that successfully demonstrate positive outcomes are measured and documented, they can be scaled or replicated in other contexts.

Informed Policy Development

Meaningful data serves as a foundation for developing policies that effectively address childhood trauma. Policymakers require solid evidence to advocate for funding, resources, and structural changes that support at-risk children and families. By utilizing data-driven insights, stakeholders can advocate for reforms that promote protective factors and resilience-building within communities.

Hearing Bill Gates speak in 1983 was a pivotal moment in my career, particularly as I began to work in the field of designing decision-making systems. His vision of the future of data systems resonated deeply with me, especially his comparison of these systems to the human central nervous system. Gates articulated a compelling future where information would be delivered precisely and efficiently, akin to how our nervous system communicates with various parts of our body—only sending signals to where they're needed. This principle of targeted information delivery not only enhances efficiency but also minimizes the noise and clutter often associated with data overload.

Inspired by Gates's insights, I firmly believe that the systems we develop must emulate this biological model. Future decision-making systems should prioritize relevance and precision, ensuring that users receive the right information at the right time, tailored to their specific needs and contexts. This not only reflects the elegance of nature's design but aligns with the growing demands of an increasingly complex world, where clarity and efficiency are paramount.

By adopting this approach, we can develop more intuitive and re-sponsive systems that enable individuals and organizations to make well-informed decisions without the distraction of superfluous data. Initially, however, it is imperative to monitor and analyze an extensive range of storytelling metrics. This will allow us to address childhood trauma effectively, supported by data, and ready to identify areas for enhanced support, refine preventative measures, and ultimately achieve improved outcomes.

CHAPTER TWENTY-SEVEN

Enhancing Support for Children

"The most powerful force for a child's development is the everyday magic of ordinary, loving human connection."

–Dr. Bruce Perry

WHEN CONSIDERING WAYS TO improve support for children, it is important to explore comprehensive methods that can promote healthy development from infancy. While there are almost endless ways to enhance support for children, this chapter explores three distinct yet interconnected dimensions of support: the foundational principles found in Norway's approach to nurturing children and the transformative power of teachers and social workers in addressing childhood trauma. By examining these cultural practices and educational and support strategies, we can glean important insights about how to better support American mothers and their children during critical developmental periods.

Together, these perspectives highlight the multifaceted nature of nurturing children, underscoring the importance of both parental support and the educational landscape in shaping resilient future generations.

Raising Children Like Vikings

Norway's focused approach to raising healthy children from birth offers valuable insights that could significantly benefit American mothers. In Norway, the government prioritizes maternal and child health, providing robust support systems designed to foster healthy development from infancy. This includes access to comprehensive prenatal and postnatal care, parental leave policies that allow parents to bond with their newborns, and educational programs that emphasize the significance of attachment and responsive caregiving. By prioritizing these elements, Norwegian society recognizes that the earliest days of a child's life are crucial for establishing the foundation for lifelong health and resilience.

One of the key aspects of Norway's system is its emphasis on parental education about the importance of early attachment. New parents receive guidance not only on the physical needs of their infants but also on the critical emotional and relational components necessary for healthy development. This includes understanding the impact of consistent, nurturing interactions during the first few months of life, which are essential for forming secure attachments. By instilling these values in parents, Norway equips them with the knowledge and confidence to foster environments that nurture their children's emotional well-being.

Further, Nordic mothers of newborns benefit from extensive government support aimed at ensuring their well-being and that of their infants. One crucial form of assistance is through healthcare programs like Medicaid, which covers prenatal care, labor and delivery, as well as postnatal check-ups. This access to vital medical services helps mothers during and after pregnancy.

Additionally, programs such as Women, Infants, and Children (WIC) offer nutritional support, providing healthy food options and education to ensure that mothers can nourish themselves and their babies effectively. Financial assistance programs like Temporary Assistance for Needy Families (TANF) also provide cash benefits to help families meet essential needs during the early stages of parenting.

Moreover, the federal Family and Medical Leave Act (FMLA) allows eligible mothers to take time off work to care for their newborns without the risk of losing their jobs. This policy empowers mothers to bond with their children and recover from childbirth, ultimately promoting maternal and infant health.

Child Welfare Systems

Nordic countries—such as Sweden, Norway, Denmark, Finland, and Iceland—are recognized for their robust welfare systems that prioritize early childhood development, parental support, and mental health services. These comprehensive systems help mitigate the effects of childhood trauma and reduce the prevalence of neglect and abuse. In contrast, the United States often lacks such extensive social safety nets, making support less accessible.

Cultural Attitudes

The cultural focus on collectivism, social responsibility, and community support in Nordic countries fosters more nurturing environments for children. This collective ethos can lead to lower rates of childhood trauma, as families often receive more assistance in challenging times. In comparison, the individualistic norms prevalent in the US can lead to increased parental stress and isolation, potentially escalating the risk of trauma for children.

Impact of Policies

Studies consistently show that Nordic nations generally experience lower rates of child poverty, better parental leave policies, and higher levels of public investment in early childhood education. These factors correlate with healthier developmental outcomes for children, resulting in reduced incidences of trauma. The US, despite its wealth, faces higher rates of child poverty and inconsistent access to support services, which can deepen the risks associated with childhood trauma.

Research Findings

Various studies highlight that while childhood trauma is a universal concern, its manifestations and prevalence can differ notably based on social and cultural contexts. Reports indicate that adverse childhood experiences (ACEs) are present in both regions, but the specific rates of abuse, neglect, and household dysfunction tend to be lower in Nordic countries compared to those in the United States.

In conclusion, while childhood trauma exists in all societies, Nordic countries demonstrate lower prevalence rates due to favorable factors such as social welfare, cultural values, and robust parenting support. By examining and adopting some practices from our Nordic neighbors, we can enhance the well-being of our children and foster healthier environments for their growth.

Transformative Teachers

Of all the potential solutions and improvements discussed throughout this book, it is the profound impact that teachers can have on addressing and mitigating childhood trauma that resonates most deeply in my mind and heart. These dedicated individuals stand as pillars of hope within our communities, endowed with the unique ability to transform lives through their compassion, leadership, and understanding. Teachers possess the rare opportunity not only to educate but also to heal, making them the key to unlocking a brighter future for our children. Their transformative influence may be the most impactful vehicle through which to address the epidemic of childhood trauma, paving the way toward a healthier, more resilient society.

Teachers play an essential role in our society. They stand at the frontline, not simply imparting knowledge, but possess the potential to nurture the hearts and minds of our children, many of whom carry the unspoken burdens of childhood trauma. As we reach the conclusion of *Greater Than Gravity*, it is imperative to spotlight these silent warriors and their infinite potential in the face of adversity.

Yet, we must acknowledge the undeniable truth: asking teachers to bear the weight of the world—including the healing of childhood trauma—is both unfair and unrealistic. Our educators are already under tremendous pressure, navigating the dual challenges of overwork and under-compensation in institutions that often overlook their invaluable contributions. A widely cited statistic that illustrates the issue of teacher underemployment comes from the Economic Policy Institute (EPI). According to their analysis, published in 2020, "Teachers earn about 19% less than similarly educated professionals."[118] This pay disparity highlights the financial challenges faced by educators, reinforcing the notion that teachers are undercompensated relative to their qualifications and the important roles they play in society. They work tirelessly with minimal resources while trying to provide their students with a nurturing environment that extends beyond academics. If we are to ask more from teachers, we should begin that discussion by committing to increase teachers' pay and training in accordance with their importance and their education.

They are often the closest, most consistent adults in a child's life beyond their guardians and are in a unique position to bridge the gap where parental support may falter. As my wife, Emilie, discovered during her tenure in a low-income district, the need for connection, compassion, and understanding stretches far beyond textbooks and tests. She spent countless nights worrying about her students—not merely their academic challenges but their emotional and social ones, clear signs of trauma masked behind classroom behaviors. Emilie embodied the essence of education; she intuitively recognized what these children needed most: love, attention, and an advocate in their corner.

Her experience is echoed by my brother, Jamie, who served as a special education teacher before becoming a principal. Time and again, I witnessed the power of his dedication. During field trips, he would prepare additional lunches because he understood that many of his students lacked the basic nourishment that should be a given. More importantly, he led his students in prayer, embodying the care and familial bond they so desperately craved. These actions fostered connection and trust.

As troubling as it is to admit, this approach begs the question: How can we place the onus of healing childhood trauma upon educators who already face overwhelming challenges? The answer lies not in expecting teachers to be saviors, but in empowering them with the tools, training, compensation, and support necessary to excel in this vital role.

To make transformative strides, we must invest in a new generation of trauma-informed educators. This involves retraining existing teachers and fostering a culture that understands and addresses the root causes of trauma. Enhanced educational models should include collaborations with mental health professionals, community outreach programs, and curriculum techniques that address emotional literacy. Equipping teachers with the understanding of childhood trauma will enable them to recognize warning signs and respond compassionately, creating safer learning environments for their students.

Such initiatives would be particularly impactful in alternative schools where the majority of students grapple with neglect, abuse, and dysfunctional home lives. In these vulnerable settings, teachers can serve as advocates and allies, helping to usher in a wave of healing. Imagine classrooms where trauma-informed practices are embedded into every lesson and interaction, where each child is seen, heard, and valued. This is not just a dream; it is a necessity.

Teachers play a critical role in children's lives as healers. We must advocate for appropriate compensation reflective of their immense responsibility, particularly including the increase in skill I propose. When teachers thrive, they will be better equipped to nurture our children, fostering resilience and hope in the face of trauma. We cannot ignore that many are already making incredible sacrifices for their students; let us not ask them to carry this burden alone. Instead, let us empower them to lead with love, understanding, and insight.

As we look toward a future where childhood trauma is no longer an epidemic, it is the teachers who will carry the torch of change. Let us support them unconditionally, rallying together to create classrooms filled with both knowledge and compassion. While we can't erase the past, we can cultivate a present and future where every child has access to the love and support they so desperately need—a future where the weight of trauma is lifted, and the light of possibility shines brightly. In the heart of every educator lies the capacity to change lives, and it is our collective duty to ensure they have the resources and support they deserve to turn that potential into reality.

It is my opinion, one that is shared by Dr. Glenn Schiraldi, that properly trained teachers in Trauma Responsive care can teach students about trauma, its consequences, principles of recovery, and treatment resources.

Transformational Social Workers: The Frontline Warriors Against Childhood Trauma

In addressing the epidemic of childhood trauma, we cannot overlook the critical role of the 750,000 social workers across America who stand at the intersection of suffering and healing. These dedicated professionals represent an army of potential change agents whose daily work brings them face-to-face with the aftermath of childhood trauma. Yet paradoxically, while nearly every client they encounter carries the weight of adverse childhood experiences, most social workers receive minimal formal education about trauma's profound neurobiological impacts and evidence-based approaches to healing.

This disconnect between the prevalence of trauma in clinical practice and the preparedness to address it creates a significant gap in our collective response to this crisis. As we've explored the Nordic model of child welfare and the transformative potential of trauma-informed educators, we must now turn our attention to empowering social workers in America as essential partners in this revolution.

The Untapped Potential

Social workers possess a unique vantage point in our society. They witness the human consequences of trauma across multiple domains—from child welfare and schools to healthcare systems and criminal justice. They work with individuals at their most vulnerable moments, often serving as the first point of professional contact for those struggling with trauma's effects. This positioning grants them unprecedented opportunities to interrupt cycles of trauma that might otherwise perpetuate through generations.

Unlike many professions, social work already embraces a holistic perspective that considers individuals within their environmental context. The profession's foundational "person-in-environment" framework naturally aligns with trauma-informed principles. Social workers understand that behavior doesn't occur in isolation but emerges from complex interactions between personal history, biology, relationships, and social systems.

What they often lack, however, is specific knowledge about how trauma literally reshapes the developing brain and nervous system, creating adaptive patterns that often manifest as the very "problems" clients present with in treatment. Without this understanding, even the most compassionate social workers may inadvertently focus on managing symptoms rather than addressing root causes.

Activating the Warriors

To fulfill their potential as transformational agents in addressing childhood trauma, social workers need both knowledge and tools. This begins with fundamental neurobiological literacy—understanding the science behind trauma's effects on brain development, stress response systems, and attachment patterns.

Social workers must learn to recognize the subtle signs of trauma that often hide behind diagnostic labels like depression, anxiety, ADHD, or conduct disorder. They need skill in distinguishing between symptoms and adaptations—seeing challenging behaviors not as problems to be eliminated but as solutions a person developed to survive overwhelming circumstances.

Beyond recognition, social workers require practical approaches for addressing trauma effectively. This includes methods for creating safety, building regulation skills, processing traumatic memories, fostering healthy attachment, and promoting post-traumatic growth. They also need guidance on preventing secondary trauma and maintaining their own well-being while doing this demanding work.

Most importantly, social workers need to be equipped as systems-change agents who can transform not just individual lives but the very institutions that often perpetuate trauma. This means developing skills in advocacy, education, and policy development that allow them to create trauma-responsive environments wherever they work.

A Call for Educational Reform

The gap between what social workers need to know about trauma and what they're typically taught represents a critical failure in professional preparation. Most Bachelor's and Master's programs in Social Work include minimal required coursework specifically addressing trauma, despite its prevalence among the populations social workers serve.

This educational oversight must be addressed through comprehensive curriculum reform. Every accredited social work program should require:

1. Foundational courses on trauma's neurobiological, psychological, and social impacts

2. Skill-based training in evidence-based trauma intervention models

3. Practical experience working with trauma survivors under trauma-informed supervision

4. Instruction on secondary trauma prevention and professional self-care

5. Training in trauma-informed organizational development and systems change

The Council on Social Work Education (CSWE), which accredits social work programs nationwide, must elevate trauma competence to a core educational requirement rather than an optional specialization. State licensing boards should similarly require demonstrated trauma knowledge for licensure and ongoing professional development.

Until such systemic changes occur, agencies employing social workers must invest in comprehensive trauma training for their staff. This investment isn't merely ethical—it's economically sound, as trauma-informed approaches have been shown to improve client outcomes, reduce staff turnover, and enhance organizational effectiveness.

The Social Worker as a Transformation Agent

What might social work practice look like when fully informed by trauma knowledge? Consider these transformational approaches:

In Child Welfare: Rather than focusing exclusively on safety and permanency, trauma-informed child protection workers recognize that removal from an unsafe home, while sometimes necessary, can itself be traumatic. They work to minimize additional trauma during investigations and placements, support birth parents in healing their own trauma, and ensure foster parents understand trauma's impacts on children's behavior and attachment.

In Schools: School social workers become bridges between educational and mental health systems, helping teachers understand students' behavioral challenges through a trauma lens. They implement group interventions that build regulation skills, advocate for discipline policies that avoid re-traumatization, and create spaces where students can safely process difficult experiences.

In Healthcare: Medical social workers recognize the connections between childhood trauma and physical health concerns like chronic pain, autoimmune disorders, and substance use. They advocate for routine trauma screening, connect patients with appropriate mental health resources, and educate medical staff about trauma-sensitive approaches to care.

In Mental Health: Clinical social workers move beyond symptom management to address the underlying dysregulation caused by trauma. They create safety first, build regulation skills before attempting insight-oriented work, and recognize that the therapeutic relationship itself is a primary healing mechanism for attachment wounds.

In Criminal Justice: Forensic social workers help courts understand the role trauma plays in criminal behavior, advocate for rehabilitation rather than punishment, and implement trauma-responsive approaches within correctional settings that support healing rather than further traumatization.

A Personal & Professional Commitment

To the social workers reading these words: Your role in addressing childhood trauma is not a burden, it is a privilege. You stand at a unique crossroads where suffering can be transformed into healing, where generational cycles can be interrupted, and where the most vulnerable members of our society can find voice and validation.

This work will demand much from you—your compassion, your creativity, your courage, and your commitment to your own well-being. It will require you to confront systems that perpetuate harm while maintaining hope in the possibility of change. It will ask you to hold space for unbearable pain while believing in unimaginable resilience.

The path of the transformational social worker isn't easy, but it offers something precious: the opportunity to participate in not just managing problems, but delivering profound healing. Every time you help a client understand that their symptoms make sense in the context of their history, every time you create safety for someone who has known only danger, every time you bear witness to someone's story with unwavering presence—you are engaging in sacred work.

At United Against Childhood Trauma, we recognize social workers as essential partners in our mission. We are committed to supporting your professional development through resources, training, and advocacy for the systemic changes needed to enhance your effectiveness. Together, we can transform not just individual lives, but entire communities affected by childhood trauma.

As we envision a future where childhood trauma no longer casts such a long shadow over human potential, we see social workers standing at the forefront of this transformation—not as lone warriors, but as leaders of a coordinated response that spans families, schools, healthcare systems, and communities. By activating and equipping this powerful workforce, we multiply our capacity to create change on a scale commensurate with the challenge we face.

The 750,000 social workers across America represent an untapped resource of immense potential in our fight against childhood trauma. When properly trained, supported, and valued, these professionals can fundamentally alter the landscape of trauma in our society, creating ripples of healing that extend far beyond individual interventions to transform our collective future.

CHAPTER TWENTY-EIGHT

Rewiring the Brain

From Fear to Freedom Through Neuroscience

"The brain is like a muscle. The more you practice a new way of thinking, the stronger those neural pathways become."

–Dr. Richard Davidson

OVER THE YEARS, AS I encountered concepts like manifestation, visualization, and mindfulness, I dismissed them as "new age fluff"—feel-good ideas without scientific merit. As an engineer and businessman who built his career on data and measurable results, I had little patience for what seemed like nonsensical thinking. However, my recent journey of understanding childhood trauma, coupled with groundbreaking neuroscience research, has transformed my perspective. What I once viewed as "woo woo" nonsense turns out to have a solid, profound foundation in brain science.

The revelation came while researching for *Greater Than Gravity* and reading Dr. James Doty's work *Into the Magic Shop*.[119] Suddenly, the pieces began falling into place—the neuroscience of trauma, the power of focused attention, and the brain's remarkable capacity for change all converged to illuminate what I now see as a path forward for trauma survivors. This explores how our nervous system responds to trauma, why many survivors remain stuck in patterns of fear and negativity, and most importantly, how we can rewire these responses through scientifically validated approaches.

Imagine your brain as a sophisticated radio receiver, constantly tuned to different frequencies that broadcast various mental and emotional states. This radio primarily operates on two main channels: the Sympathetic Nervous System (SNS), our "emergency broadcast" channel, and the Parasympathetic Nervous System (PNS), our "safety and connection" channel.

The SNS channel broadcasts emergency alerts, which triggers our fight-or-flight response, when we perceive danger. It increases our heart rate, tenses muscles, and floods our system with stress hormones like cortisol and adrenaline. You know, like when we see Bigfoot. This channel evolved to keep us alive in times of genuine threat. But being on this channel limits our ability to feel, be creative, and to learn and grow.

In contrast, the PNS channel plays songs of safety and connection. When tuned to this frequency, our body relaxes, our heart rate steadies, and our mind opens to possibilities rather than threats. This is where we can access creativity, form meaningful connections, and experience joy.

For those who haven't experienced significant trauma, the brain's radio can easily switch between these stations automatically when appropriate, and as needed. However, childhood trauma can, and often does leave the dial stuck on the emergency channel, creating a constant state of hypervigilance and fear.

Here is the science behind the struggle. When a child experiences trauma, their brain does exactly what it's designed to do—it adapts for survival. The amygdala, our brain's threat detection center, becomes hyperactive, while the prefrontal cortex, responsible for rational thinking and emotional regulation, may become under-stimulated. This isn't a malfunction; it's the brain's way of prioritizing survival.

Dr. Bruce Perry's research shows that chronic trauma exposure during childhood can alter the physical structure of the brain, leading to an oversensitive threat detection system.[120] The brain becomes like a radio that's been modified to amplify emergency broadcasts while muting signals of safety and opportunity.

This helps explain why many trauma survivors report being constantly on edge, expecting disaster around every corner. Their brain's radio is perpetually tuned to a station that broadcasts messages like "You're not enough," "You don't deserve happiness," or "Something bad is about to happen." And sadly, the sufferer begins to believe this narrative. These aren't character flaws or signs of weakness—they're the result of neurobiological adaptations to early adversity.

When the Emergency Channel Won't Stop Broadcasting

Being stuck in sympathetic nervous system (SNS) dominance—that emergency broadcast channel—is like living with an alarm that never stops ringing. Research shows that when our SNS remains chronically activated, it doesn't just create psychological distress; it generates very real physical pain and suffering. Dr. Bessel van der Kolk's research reveals that people with chronic SNS activation often experience persistent muscle tension, headaches, digestive issues, and a host of other physical symptoms that can feel mystifying to both patients and doctors.[17]

But why does this happen? When our nervous system remains stuck in "danger mode," it floods our body with stress hormones like cortisol and adrenaline. These chemicals are meant for short-term emergency responses—like escaping that metaphorical Bigfoot in the woods. They're not meant to course through our system continuously. When they do, they create inflammation, disrupt our sleep patterns, and even change how our brain processes pain signals.

This constant state of physiological stress does something else particularly insidious: it amplifies the volume of negative thoughts and memories. The brain becomes like a radio stuck between stations, creating a kind of "neural static" that can manifest as anxiety, depression, or a pervasive sense of impending doom. The internal messages become relentless: "You're not safe," "Something bad is about to happen," "You'll never be good enough."

Is it any wonder, then, that so many trauma survivors turn to alcohol, drugs, or other addictive behaviors to find relief? These substances can temporarily quiet the emergency broadcast—providing a brief respite from the constant neural static and physical discomfort. They act as a temporary volume knob, turning down the intensity of both physical pain and emotional anguish.

In fact, the original ACEs study report that those with 4+ ACEs are 1,132% more likely to use illegal intravenous drugs.[8] This isn't about moral failing or lack of willpower—it's about attempting to regulate an overactive nervous system the only way they know how. The same neural mechanisms that keep the radio stuck on the emergency channel can make these coping mechanisms feel like the only path to peace.

This also explains why traditional addiction treatment often falls short when it doesn't address the underlying trauma keeping the nervous system stuck in emergency mode. Just as treating a fever without addressing the underlying infection won't lead to true healing, addressing addiction without helping to regulate the nervous system often results in a cycle of relapse.

Understanding this biological basis for addiction can help shift our perspective from judgment to compassion. It also points toward more effective solutions: if we can help trauma survivors learn to switch their neural radio station—through methods like gratitude practice, mindfulness, journaling, and other nervous system regulation techniques—we might be able to reduce their need for chemical regulation of their internal state.

The Power of Gratitude: A Neurobiological Game-Changer

Perhaps no story better illustrates the transformative power of shifting our nervous system's "radio station" than a cherished memory from my childhood on May Avenue. We were poor—genuinely poor—with a single lightbulb that we would unscrew and carry from room to room because we couldn't afford another. Each night, as we gathered to move the bulb upstairs for bedtime, my mother would transform what could have been a moment of shame or resentment into something magical.

"We have a lightbulb!" she would exclaim, leading us up the dark stairs. "Do you know how lucky we are to have a lightbulb? How many families don't have a light bulb? Thank you, Jesus, for our light bulb!" This gratitude over our one lightbulb repeated every night.

What I now understand, through the lens of neuroscience, is that my mother was intuitively practicing what researchers call "neural reframing." Instead of allowing our brains to attune to the frequency of lack and deprivation—which would activate our threat response system (SNS)—she was actively guiding us to tune into gratitude, which engages the parasympathetic nervous system (PNS) and creates entirely different neural patterns. Did she know what she was doing? Oh, how I'd love one more talk with her.

Recent studies using functional MRI scans show that expressing gratitude activates areas in the brain associated with dopamine and serotonin production—our natural "feel-good" neurotransmitters. Dr. Andrew Huberman's research at Stanford has demonstrated that practicing gratitude, especially in challenging circumstances, can:

- Reduce activity in the amygdala, our brain's threat-detection center

- Increase activity in the medial prefrontal cortex, associated with understanding others' perspectives and empathy

- Strengthen neural pathways associated with positive expectation and resilience

My Mother's Manifestation: A Lesson in Possibility

Neural reframing through gratitude illuminates another powerful story from my childhood. In my memoir, *The Kite That Couldn't Fly*, I recounted entering the grand kite contest. Despite our poverty and limited resources, my mother helped me create a beautiful kite adorned with the biblical image of Jacob's Ladder.

Each night, as we worked on the kite, I would anxiously ask her where we would put the trophy when I won. Notice I didn't say "if"—because my mother never allowed that possibility into our consciousness. She would respond, with unwavering certainty, "We'll put that giant trophy right on top of the TV where all the neighbors can see it." I would ask that question of my mother multiple times each night.

I needed to hear that answer, which she patiently delivered each time, with conviction.

What I now understand is that my mother wasn't just being optimistic—she was actively helping to tune my brain's radio to a different frequency. Instead of the fear-based station that poverty and trauma had set as my default, she was teaching me to access the frequency of possibility and achievement.

That kite never did fly—but it won first place for beauty and creativity. My mother had manifested this victory, not through magic, but through her deep understanding of how to shift a child's perspective from limitation to possibility. Looking back, these sublime lessons have served me well my entire life.

We are learning more every day about the neuroscience of transformation. Recent research provides compelling evidence for our ability to rewire trauma responses. Studies using functional MRI scans show that practices like mindfulness, meditation, and gratitude can actually change the structure and function of key brain regions involved in emotion regulation and stress response.

Dr. Richard Davidson's groundbreaking work[121] at the University of Wisconsin-Madison demonstrates that regular meditation practice can:

- Reduce activity in the amygdala (our fear center)

- Strengthen the prefrontal cortex (our rational thinking center)

- Increase production of GABA (a neurotransmitter that promotes calm and well-being)

These changes aren't mystical—they're measurable alterations in brain structure and function. When we consistently practice tuning our brain's radio to the frequency of safety and possibility, we create new neural pathways that make it easier to access these states in the future.

There are practical steps we can take to change the radio station. The journey from fear to freedom is possible when we leverage our understanding of neuroscience.

1. **Awareness:** Learn to recognize when you're stuck on the "emergency broadcast" channel. Physical symptoms like rapid heartbeat, shallow breathing, or muscle tension are clear signals.
2. **Breath Work:** Deep, slow breathing activates the vagus nerve, which helps switch from SNS to PNS dominance. This isn't mystical—it's a direct biological mechanism for changing your nervous system state.
3. **Gratitude Practice:** As I learned from my mother, and as my friend Trent discovered in his healing journey, gratitude isn't just positive thinking—it's a powerful tool for rewiring the brain. Research shows that regular gratitude practice increases dopamine and serotonin production, naturally countering the stress hormones of trauma.
4. **Visualization:** When we visualize positive outcomes while in a calm state, we create new neural pathways that make those outcomes more accessible. This isn't manifestation magic—it's neuroplasticity in action.
5. **Progressive Exposure:** Gradually exposing yourself to safe situations that trigger anxiety, while maintaining awareness of your nervous system state, helps recalibrate your threat detection system.

Understanding the neuroscience behind trauma responses offers hope and validation. You're not broken, and you're not stuck forever on the emergency broadcast channel. Your brain adapted to help you survive, and with understanding and practice, it can adapt again to help you thrive.

The path forward isn't about denying your past or forcing positive thinking. It's about understanding how your nervous system works and learning to guide it toward states of safety and connection. This isn't new age philosophy—it's neuroscience. And while the journey may be challenging, knowing that change is physically possible can provide the hope needed to begin.

Remember: Your brain's radio may be stuck on the fear frequency, but you have the power to change the station. Just as my mother taught me to tune into possibility through gratitude and vision, and as Trent discovered through his own practice, you can learn to access frequencies of hope, connection, and growth.

The science is clear: your brain can change. The question is, are you ready to turn the dial?

CHAPTER TWENTY-NINE

Beyond Trauma-Informed

The Revolution in How We Classify & Address Childhood Trauma

"The difference between trauma-informed and trauma-responsive is the difference between accommodation and transformation. It's the difference between knowing and doing."

–Michael Menard

AS WE STAND AT the precipice of a national awakening to childhood trauma's devastating impact, we face a critical challenge that threatens to undermine our entire movement: the linguistic chaos surrounding what it means to be "trauma-informed." This seemingly academic distinction represents one of the most urgent obstacles to our mission of ending childhood trauma in America.

Walk into any conference on social services, education, healthcare, or corporate wellness, and you'll hear the phrase "trauma-informed" used to describe everything from basic awareness training to comprehensive healing programs. A hospital that screens for adverse childhood experiences calls itself trauma-informed. So does a school that simply trains teachers to recognize trauma symptoms. Meanwhile, a corporate wellness program that mentions trauma in employee orientations claims the same designation as a residential treatment facility providing intensive trauma therapy.

This linguistic imprecision isn't just semantics—it's sabotaging our national response to what we now know is the leading cause of death in America.

The Devastating Cost of Confusion

When everything is "trauma-informed," nothing truly is. I have documented throughout this book that childhood trauma affects 180 million American adults, drives the majority of addiction and suicide cases, and costs our economy $14.1 trillion annually. Yet organizations across every sector claim trauma-informed status without any standardized criteria for what that actually means.

The consequences extend far beyond administrative confusion. When organizations claim trauma-informed status without systematic practices to prevent re-traumatization or promote healing, they're not just ineffective—they're often harmful. A "trauma-informed" school that still relies on suspension and punishment may actually worsen outcomes for traumatized students. A "trauma-informed" workplace that provides awareness training but maintains authoritarian management practices creates cognitive dissonance that undermines trust and safety.

Most tragically, it betrays trauma survivors. When someone seeks help from a "trauma-informed" organization, they have no way to know whether they'll encounter someone who understands trauma's neurobiological impact and responds accordingly, or someone who attended a workshop once and learned to ask, "What happened to you?" without any capacity for meaningful intervention.

The Four-Tier Revolution

Through extensive research and field testing across corporate, educational, and faith-based organizations, United Against Childhood Trauma (UACT) has developed a standardized classification system that distinguishes between levels of trauma competency. This framework provides the clarity our movement desperately needs to measure progress, allocate resources effectively, and hold organizations accountable for their claims.

Trauma-Unaware: "We Don't Have a Trauma Problem Here"

These organizations operate under the assumption that people's problems stem primarily from personal failures or poor choices. They rely heavily on punitive approaches, zero-tolerance policies, and authoritarian leadership. When confronted with behavioral or performance issues, their response is discipline and consequences rather than understanding and support.

The language reveals their mindset: "They just need more discipline," "People need to take personal responsibility," and "We can't coddle everyone." These aren't necessarily bad people, but they operate from a worldview that predates our understanding of trauma's neurobiological impact.

Trauma-Aware: "Trauma Exists, But We're Not Sure What to Do"

Organizations at this level recognize that trauma affects people but lack systematic approaches to address it. They have good intentions and may have provided basic training, but their responses remain inconsistent and reactive. Staff members may understand trauma's impact intellectually but struggle to translate that knowledge into effective practice.

These organizations often experience frustration because their caring intentions don't translate into measurable improvements. They know they should respond differently to trauma-affected individuals but lack the tools, training, and systematic approaches to do so effectively.

Trauma-Informed: "We Understand and Have Systematic Responses"

This is where most organizations aspire to be, and it represents a significant achievement. True trauma-informed organizations have implemented comprehensive policies, provided systematic training, and modified their environments to prevent re-traumatization. They operate from the six key principles: safety, trustworthiness, peer support, collaboration, empowerment, and attention to cultural issues.

However—and this is crucial—trauma-informed organizations focus primarily on avoiding harm rather than actively promoting healing. They ask, "What happened to you?" instead of "What's wrong with you?" They create safe environments and respond empathetically to trauma-related behaviors. But they don't necessarily provide interventions that help people heal from trauma's effects or prevent it.

Trauma-Responsive: "We Don't Just Understand—We Actively Heal and Prevent"

Trauma-responsive organizations go beyond preventing re-traumatization to actively promoting healing and post-traumatic growth. They provide trauma-specific interventions, measure healing outcomes, and integrate recovery into their core mission. These organizations don't just accommodate trauma—they help people overcome it and prevent it for future generations.

The distinction is profound. A trauma-informed school creates safe spaces and responds empathetically when students have trauma reactions. A trauma-responsive school does all of that *plus* provides on-site counseling, teaches emotional regulation skills, implements somatic interventions, and measures students' healing progress over time.

The Critical Divide: Knowing vs. Doing

The most important boundary in our classification system falls between trauma-informed and trauma-responsive. This isn't just an academic distinction—it represents the difference between accommodation and transformation, between knowing about the trauma epidemic and actually addressing it.

Trauma-informed approaches ask: How can we avoid making things worse? Trauma-responsive approaches ask: How can we make things better?

Trauma-informed organizations create safety. Trauma-responsive organizations create healing.

Trauma-informed practices prevent re-traumatization. Trauma-responsive practices promote post-traumatic growth.

Consider the difference in a corporate setting. A trauma-informed workplace might train managers to recognize signs of trauma, create employee assistance programs, and modify performance reviews to account for trauma's effects. A trauma-responsive workplace does all of that plus provides on-site trauma therapy, implements mindfulness and somatic programs, measures employees' resilience and well-being over time, and actively promotes healing through evidence-based interventions.

Both approaches have value, but only one actively addresses the root causes of the trauma epidemic we've documented throughout this book. In our current crisis—where 1,401 Americans die daily from trauma-related causes—accommodation alone is insufficient. We need healing.

The Business Case for Transformation

Beyond moral imperatives, standardized trauma classifications provide concrete organizational benefits that align with UACT's economic arguments:

For Funders and Policymakers: Clear criteria for evaluating grant applications and contract awards. No more funding "trauma-informed" programs that provide minimal training while ignoring those offering comprehensive healing services. When we're hemorrhaging $14.1 trillion annually to trauma's effects, resource allocation must be strategic.

For Organizations: Honest assessment tools that reveal current capacity and create roadmaps for improvement. Clear benchmarks for measuring progress and demonstrating impact to stakeholders. Remember: Every dollar invested in trauma prevention saves $191 in future costs.

For Individuals Seeking Services: Transparent information about what level of trauma competency they can expect. The difference between a trauma-aware counselor who recognizes trauma symptoms and a trauma-responsive therapist who provides evidence-based trauma treatment could be the difference between continued suffering and genuine healing.

For Communities: Strategic resource allocation based on actual capacity rather than claimed competency. The ability to identify gaps in trauma-responsive services and prioritize development accordingly.

Measuring What Matters

Each classification level requires different metrics that align with our broader mission to track progress against the trauma epidemic. Trauma-aware organizations might track staff training completion and policy modifications. Trauma-informed organizations measure re-traumatization incidents, environmental safety indicators, and staff retention.

Trauma-responsive organizations focus on healing outcomes: reduced PTSD symptoms, increased resilience scores, improved life functioning, and post-traumatic growth indicators. This measurement hierarchy prevents organizations from gaming the system by focusing on inputs rather than outcomes—a crucial distinction when addressing a crisis of this magnitude.

A truly trauma-responsive organization must demonstrate that people are actually healing, not just that staff attended training sessions. When we're confronting the leading cause of death in America, we need accountability for results, not just intentions.

Implementation Roadmap

Organizations cannot leap from trauma unaware to trauma responsive overnight. The transformation requires systematic progression through each level, much like the comprehensive approach for which we've advocated throughout this book for addressing the trauma epidemic:

Phase 1: Becoming Trauma-Aware

- Leadership education on trauma's prevalence and impact

- Basic staff training on trauma recognition

- Initial policy review to identify most harmful practices

- Beginning to track relevant metrics

Phase 2: Becoming Trauma-Informed

- Comprehensive implementation of trauma-informed principles

- Systematic staff training across all levels

- Policy and procedure overhaul

- Environmental modifications to enhance safety

- Regular measurement and feedback systems

Phase 3: Becoming Trauma-Responsive

- Integration of trauma-specific healing interventions

- Partnership with trauma treatment specialists

- Outcome measurement focused on healing and growth

- Community collaboration and systems change efforts

The timeline matters because cultural transformation cannot be rushed. Organizations that attempt to skip levels often experience staff resistance, implementation failures, and ultimate regression to previous practices—outcomes we cannot afford when confronting a crisis of this scope.

The Call to Standardization

The trauma epidemic will not be solved by good intentions or surface-level awareness. It requires systematic, evidence-based approaches that actively promote healing. Our current practice of calling everything "trauma-informed" obscures the critical difference between organizations that accommodate trauma and those that heal it.

We call on professional associations, accrediting bodies, funding organizations, and government agencies to adopt standardized trauma classifications. The framework exists. The research supporting it is robust. What we need now is the collective will to implement standards that distinguish between knowing about trauma and doing something *effective* about it.

This standardization is not an abstract academic exercise—it's a practical necessity for our movement's success. When we're fighting to save 1,401 lives daily and prevent 1.783 billion years of stolen human potential, precision in our language and clarity in our classifications become matters of life and death.

Your Role in the Revolution

As members of United Against Childhood Trauma, each of us has a responsibility to advance this classification revolution:

Demand Clarity: When organizations claim to be trauma-informed, ask specific questions about their practices. What training have staff received? What policies have been modified? What healing interventions do they provide? What outcomes do they measure?

Advocate for Standards: Push professional associations, accrediting bodies, and licensing organizations in your field to adopt standardized trauma classifications. The confusion serves no one except those who prefer to hide behind vague terminology.

Assess Your Own Organization: Use the four-tier framework to honestly evaluate where your workplace, school, or community organization currently stands. Create action plans for advancing to the next level, with specific timelines and accountability measures.

Support Truly Responsive Organizations: When you have choices about where to work, where to send your children to school, or where to seek services, prioritize organizations that have achieved trauma-responsive status through measurable actions, not just proclaimed intentions.

The Dawn of Precision

We stand at a critical juncture in our movement. The awareness I've built through this book and through UACT's efforts has created momentum, but momentum without precision can dissipate into ineffectual gesturing. By demanding standardized classifications, we transform awareness into accountability and intentions into impact.

The children across America who represent those 54 million current trauma victims, and the adults who make up those 180 million trauma survivors, deserve better than semantic confusion. They deserve organizations that don't just understand their pain but actively work to heal and prevent it. That's the difference between trauma-informed and trauma-responsive. That's the difference between accommodation and transformation.

That's the difference between knowing and doing.

When everything is trauma-informed, nothing truly is. But when we implement clear standards, measure actual outcomes, and hold ourselves accountable for healing rather than just acknowledging trauma, we create the foundation for genuine transformation.

This classification revolution is not the end goal—it's the infrastructure that makes our ultimate goal achievable. By creating clarity in how we measure trauma competency, we accelerate progress toward our vision of a world where childhood trauma becomes increasingly rare and where survivors receive the healing they deserve.

The revolution begins with precision. The transformation begins with truth. And both begin with our commitment to move beyond the comfortable ambiguity of "trauma-informed" to the demanding accountability of "trauma-responsive."

Our movement's success depends on it. American children's lives depend on it. The future we're fighting to create depends on it.

The time for linguistic precision is now. The time for measured accountability is now. The time to distinguish between knowing and doing is now.

Join us in this classification revolution. Because in the fight against childhood trauma, precision saves lives.

In Memoriam

Trent's Legacy

BEFORE THIS BOOK WENT to press, I received devastating news that shattered my heart. Trent, whose powerful journey of trauma and healing you read about in these pages, left this world just days after this manuscript was completed.

Trent's story now stands as both a beacon of hope and a solemn reminder of trauma's unyielding grip. His willingness to share his struggles was an act of profound courage, intended to help others find their path toward healing. Though his own journey ended in tragedy, the impact of his openness lives on in these pages and in the lives of those he touched.

This loss reinforces what Trent named as a force "greater than gravity"—the weight that childhood trauma places on the human spirit. It is a force so powerful that even those who appear to have conquered it remain vulnerable to its pull. Trent's passing is not a failure of his recovery but a testament to how deeply these wounds can penetrate, and how vigilantly we must work to address them.

In honor of Trent's memory, I have titled this book *Greater Than Gravity*, and I dedicate my continued work to ensuring his story serves as a catalyst for the change we so desperately need. The urgency of our mission to prevent childhood trauma and support its survivors has never been more evident.

May Trent find the peace that eluded him in life, and may we find the collective will to create a world where such suffering becomes increasingly rare.

The Dawn of a New Era

A Declaration of War Against America's Hidden Killer

"The ultimate measure of a man is not where he stands in moments of comfort and convenience, but where he stands at times of challenge and controversy."

–Martin Luther King Jr.

WE STAND AT A crossroads of history. Behind us lies devastation so vast it defies comprehension—1,401 Americans dying daily from the leading cause of death in our nation, 1.783 billion years of human life stolen over the next generation, and a $14 trillion economic hemorrhage that exceeds our entire defense budget. Ahead of us stretch two divergent paths: continued complicity in preventable suffering, or the greatest humanitarian triumph in modern history.

For too long, we have normalized the abnormal. We have allowed childhood trauma—this silent assassin—to operate in the shadows, claiming more lives than cancer, heart disease, and stroke combined while remaining invisible to public consciousness. But the shadows have been illuminated. The data is irrefutable.

This is our generation's defining moment.

Just as our predecessors rose to defeat polio, slash smoking rates by 70%, and reduce HIV infections by 73%, we now face our own monumental challenge. The difference is that our enemy strikes at the very foundation of human development, warping the architecture of childhood and casting shadows across entire lifespans.

But here's what sets us apart: we possess something previous generations lacked. We have the knowledge, the tools, and the proven interventions to not just treat childhood trauma, but to prevent it entirely. We stand on the shoulders of giants like Drs. Felitti, Anda, Van der Kolk, Schiraldi, and Burke Harris, who have illuminated the path forward with scientific precision.

The question is not whether we can end childhood trauma. The question is whether we have the moral courage to act on what we know.

The Birth of a Movement: United Against Childhood Trauma

From the ashes of my family's pain—the deaths of my brothers Patrick and Adam, the decades of hidden suffering among my 13 siblings, and my own 75-year journey to understanding—has emerged something extraordinary. United Against Childhood Trauma (UACT) represents more than an organization. It is the crystallization of humanity's collective awakening to its greatest unaddressed crisis.

UACT embodies three revolutionary pillars:

Awareness: We will make childhood trauma impossible to ignore through comprehensive public education campaigns, documentary series, social media movements, and virtual reality experiences that create visceral understanding. Our goal: 50% awareness by 2030, 75% by 2035, and 95% by 2050.

Healing: We will revolutionize how we treat trauma's devastating effects by training 750,000 social workers in trauma-informed care, transforming educational systems into healing environments, and scaling proven interventions like EMDR and trauma-responsive therapy.

Prevention: We will attack trauma at its source by supporting mothers during the sacred first 60 days, implementing trauma-responsive policies in schools and communities, and creating the social infrastructure that makes childhood trauma increasingly rare.

The Mathematics of Transformation

The scope of our mission matches the magnitude of our crisis. Victory means:

- **511,427 lives saved annually** through comprehensive trauma prevention

- **1.783 billion years of human life reclaimed** over the next generation

- **$14 trillion in economic devastation prevented** through early intervention

- **Millions of families spared** the agony of losing children to suicide, substance abuse, and premature death

But the mathematics work in reverse as well. Every day we delay action costs lives. Every month of inaction costs us nearly $1.2 trillion in economic damage. The moral calculation is even starker: we are either part of the solution, or we are complicit in the continuation of America's greatest preventable tragedy.

The Call to Arms: Your Nation Needs You

This moment demands action. Each of us must step forward and declare: "Not in my community. Not to my children or grandchildren."

To Parents and Grandparents: Your children's future depends on your action today. Join UACT to ensure they grow up in communities that understand trauma and schools that heal rather than harm.

To Educators: You hold the power to transform lives daily. Become trauma-responsive. Create healing environments. Recognize that the "difficult" child is almost always a wounded child seeking safety.

To Healthcare Professionals: Every patient you see carries the potential imprint of childhood trauma. Learn to recognize it. Address root causes, not just symptoms.

To Faith Communities: Your congregations are filled with trauma survivors seeking hope and healing. Become trauma-informed sanctuaries where wounded souls find understanding, not judgment.

To Business Leaders: Your workforces carry this invisible burden, costing productivity while driving healthcare costs through the roof. Invest in trauma-responsive workplace cultures and watch both human flourishing and bottom lines improve.

To Policymakers: Childhood trauma prevention offers the highest return on investment of any public health intervention. Fund it. Prioritize it. Make it impossible for communities to ignore.

To Every American: There is no neutral ground when lives hang in the balance every single day.

A Vision of Victory

Imagine schools where every teacher understands that behavior is communication, where "difficult" children are seen as wounded children deserving compassion rather than punishment. Communities where new parents receive comprehensive support during those crucial first 60 days. Healthcare systems that address trauma at its roots rather than merely treating its symptoms decades later.

Imagine families free from the cycles of addiction, violence, and premature death that have plagued generations. Imagine the innovations, the art, the leadership, and the love that will emerge when human potential is no longer constrained by the invisible chains of unhealed childhood wounds.

This is not utopian dreaming. This is achievable reality based on proven science and demonstrated interventions. Other nations have already begun this journey. We have the roadmap. We have the tools. We need only the will.

Your Marching Orders

Immediate Action:

- Visit www.UACTNOW.com and join our movement

- Share this book with 10 people who need to understand

- Identify three ways you can make your community more trauma-informed

- Commit financial resources—every dollar invested in trauma prevention saves $191 in future costs

Ongoing Commitment:
- Become educated about trauma's signs and impacts

- Advocate for trauma-responsive policies in your workplace, school, and community

- Support trauma survivors with understanding and resources

- Vote for leaders who prioritize childhood well-being

The Final Choice

You can close this book, feel moved by the stories and statistics, perhaps share a few insights with friends, and return to your life largely unchanged. Childhood trauma will continue its silent devastation.

Or you can choose to be part of the generation that says: "This ends with us."

You can join UACT and help create the most important social movement of the 21st century. You can become part of the force that protects childhood, heals survivors, and prevents trauma before it occurs.

The children cannot save themselves. The survivors often cannot heal alone. The systems will not change without pressure. But together—united against childhood trauma—we possess the power to accomplish what no generation before us could even imagine: the end of humanity's most devastating preventable crisis.

The Shot Heard Around the World

Let this book be our generation's shot heard around the world—the moment when silence about childhood trauma ended forever, when passive acceptance transformed into active resistance, when individual awareness crystallized into collective action.

From this moment forward, let it be said that we knew the truth and acted upon it. That when faced with evidence of unprecedented suffering, we chose courage over comfort, action over apathy, hope over despair.

Let it be said that we were the generation that refused to accept preventable childhood trauma deaths. That we were the ones who looked at 54 million traumatized children and said: "Not on our watch."

The enemy is formidable, but we are stronger. The challenge is enormous, but our cause is just. The task is urgent, but our resources are sufficient.

The children are counting on us.

The survivors are trusting us.

History is watching us.

United Against Childhood Trauma, we will prevail. Not because victory is guaranteed, but because defeat is unacceptable.

The movement begins now.

Join us at www.UACTNOW.com
Together, we will save American childhood.

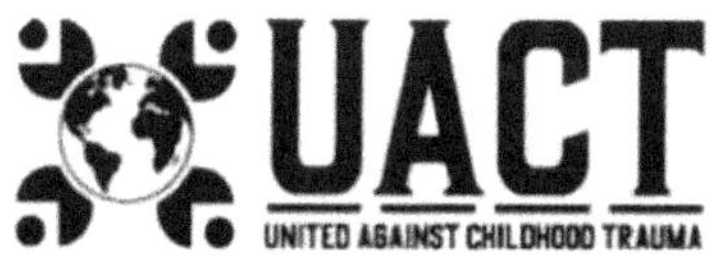

United Against Childhood Trauma. The Shot Heard Around the World.

AWARENESS | HEALING | PREVENTION

www.uactnow.com

Acknowledgments

As I reflect on the journey that has led to the creation of *Greater Than Gravity*, my heart is filled with gratitude for those who've walked alongside me, both known and unknown. This endeavor would not have been possible without the contributions—large and small—of countless individuals who believed in this mission and fueled my passion to address the silent crisis of childhood trauma.

First and foremost, to my amazing wife, Emilie: your unwavering love, emotional support, and insightful guidance have been my anchor throughout this process. I am endlessly grateful for your presence in my life. I thank you for the freedom you have given to me to chase my ideas and dreams. To my daughters—Laura, Jenna, Melissa, Anna, and Stella—I offer my heartfelt thanks. You are my greatest advisors, and I trust your instincts more than my own. Your perspectives have enriched this work more than you will ever know.

To my brothers and sisters, Jamie, Polly, David, Mary, Tim, Bill, Warren, Maria, Mark, and Ellen, thank you for sharing this journey of discovery and healing of our lives. Together, we have unveiled the complexities of childhood trauma, and your support has been a source of strength. I want to extend special gratitude to brother Jamie for his research guidance and sister Mary for walking beside me with unwavering faith and encouragement every step of the way.

To my editor, Allison Buehner, thank you for sharing your exceptional talents and insights with me throughout this journey. You possess a unique combination of being a meticulous editor and a literary expert, all while remaining a trusted friend who encouraged me to push my boundaries and strive for excellence.

I am also deeply appreciative of the friendship of Dr. Glenn Schiraldi, who I regard as the world's authority on trauma, recovery, and resilience. Your wisdom and guidance have illuminated my path.

To Kristin Trudeau, a therapist and my mentor, thank you for inspiring me to find my voice and motivating my writing in ways I never anticipated.

Thank you to Dr. Lee Long. Your insights and heartfelt stories have provided me with a lens of understanding that has been invaluable.

To the brilliant authors whose important work and words have guided me: Though I have not yet met you in person, your work has ignited my drive to write this book. Admittedly, I lack formal education on these topics, but your writings have served as the coal stoking the fire of my passion. Each of you has spoken directly to my soul, illuminating the path forward. Dr. Glenn Schiraldi, Dr. Nadine Burke Harris, and Dr. Bessel van der Kolk, thank you for sharing your knowledge and experiences. It is my hope that by connecting some of the dots between your insights and my own, I will motivate readers to join us to take the crucial steps toward healing and action.

To my friend Nate Tabler, who has been a quiet voice delivering thought-provoking comments and questions that prompt deep thinking, always with perfect timing.

To Carey Sipp and Dana Brown from PACEs Connect, two pioneers in the trauma space. Thank you for your early direction, support, and motivation.

I am grateful for everyone who has contributed to this book, shaping it into a testament of resilience and a call to awareness. May we rise together in solidarity to end the cycle of childhood trauma, for the well-being of individuals, families, and humanity as a whole.

Glossary

ACEs (Adverse Childhood Experiences) - Traumatic events that occur during childhood (ages 0-17), including abuse, neglect, and household dysfunction. Originally identified through a landmark 1998 study by Drs. Vincent Felitti and Robert Anda that revealed strong connections between childhood trauma and adult health problems.

ACEs Score - A numerical rating (0-10) based on the original ACEs assessment tool that measures the number of adverse childhood experiences a person has endured. Higher scores correlate with increased risk of mental and physical health problems. Recent research has expanded this to include up to 18 types of traumatic experiences.

Adrenaline (Epinephrine) - A stress hormone produced by the adrenal glands that triggers the fight-or-flight response. Causes increased heart rate, blood pressure, and redirects blood flow to essential muscles for survival.

Amygdala - A small, almond-shaped region in the brain that processes emotions and detects threats. In trauma survivors, the amygdala often becomes hyperactive, leading to heightened fear responses and difficulty distinguishing between real and perceived dangers.

Apoptosis - The process of programmed cell death. Chronic cortisol exposure from trauma can trigger mitochondria to self-destruct through this process.

Attachment - The emotional bond between a child and their primary caregiver, typically formed in the first year of life. Secure attachment provides a foundation for healthy development, while disrupted attachment can increase vulnerability to trauma and lead to attachment disorders.

Attachment Disorder - A condition characterized by difficulties in emotional attachments with caregivers, often resulting from early neglect or abuse. Symptoms include withdrawal from caregivers, difficulty showing affection, and problems with emotional regulation.

ATP (Adenosine Triphosphate) - The primary energy currency of cells, produced by mitochondria through cellular respiration. Essential for all cellular functions.

Bilateral Stimulation - A technique used in EMDR therapy that involves rhythmic left-right stimulation (typically eye movements) to help process traumatic memories.

Brain Fog - A cognitive symptom characterized by difficulty concentrating, memory problems, and mental fatigue, often resulting from mitochondrial dysfunction in trauma survivors.

Catatonia - An extreme version of metabolic failure seen in people with underlying mood or psychotic disorders, where individuals appear paralyzed and have severe difficulty moving or speaking.

Cellular Respiration - The process by which mitochondria convert food and oxygen into usable energy (ATP).

Child-Parent Psychotherapy (CPP) - A therapeutic approach developed by Dr. Alicia Lieberman that focuses on improving the relationship between young children and their caregivers.

Complex Trauma (C-PTSD) - Prolonged or repeated exposure to traumatic events, particularly those occurring within caregiving relationships. Unlike single-incident trauma, complex trauma typically involves multiple adverse experiences that compound over time, occurring in childhood within the primary caregiving environment.

Cortisol - A stress hormone released by the adrenal glands during the fight-or-flight response. While helpful in short-term emergencies, chronic elevation of cortisol due to ongoing trauma can damage the immune system, brain development, mitochondria, and overall health.

Developmental Adversity - A term used to describe the cumulative impact of adverse experiences during critical developmental periods, particularly the first 60 days of life.

Disintegration - The breakdown or loss of cohesion within an individual's mental, physical, spiritual, and social dimensions following trauma. This can manifest as fragmented thoughts, physical ailments, spiritual disconnection, and relationship difficulties.

Dissociation - A psychological defense mechanism where a person disconnects from their thoughts, emotions, or physical sensations during overwhelming stress. This can manifest as feeling detached from oneself or one's surroundings, or experiencing a sense of unreality.

Dysregulation - The inability to effectively regulate emotions, behaviors, or physiological responses. Common in trauma survivors due to disrupted brain development and stress response systems.

EMDR (Eye Movement Desensitization and Reprocessing) - An evidence-based therapy that uses bilateral stimulation (typically eye movements) to help process traumatic memories and reduce their emotional impact.

Emotional Neglect - A form of childhood trauma where a child's emotional needs for love, attention, and validation are consistently unmet by caregivers.

Epigenetics - The study of how environmental factors can influence gene expression without changing the DNA sequence itself. Trauma can create epigenetic changes that may be passed down through generations.

Feedback Inhibition - The body's mechanism for turning off the stress response once a threat has passed. In trauma survivors, this system often malfunctions, leading to chronic stress activation.

Fight-or-Flight Response - The body's automatic physiological reaction to perceived threats, involving the release of stress hormones and physical changes that prepare the body to either confront danger or escape from it.

Flashbacks - Intrusive, involuntary memories where a person vividly re-experiences a traumatic event as if it were happening in the present moment.

Fragmented Memories - Incomplete or disjointed memories of traumatic events. The brain protects itself from overwhelming pain by storing trauma fragments in different corners of consciousness, making it difficult to form coherent narratives.

Gut-Brain Axis - The bidirectional communication system between the gastrointestinal tract and the brain. Trauma can disrupt this connection, leading to various digestive disorders.

Hippocampus - A brain region essential for memory formation and emotional regulation. Chronic stress and elevated cortisol can cause the hippocampus to shrink, impacting learning ability and emotional processing.

HPA Axis (Hypothalamic-Pituitary-Adrenal Axis) - A complex set of interactions between the hypothalamus, pituitary gland, and adrenal glands that regulates the stress response and release of cortisol.

Hyperarousal - A state of increased physiological and psychological activation characterized by elevated heart rate, heightened alertness, and difficulty relaxing, common in trauma survivors.

Hypervigilance – A state of constant alertness and scanning for potential threats, common in trauma survivors. This heightened awareness can be exhausting and interfere with daily functioning.

Implicit Memory – Memories stored without conscious awareness, often expressed through emotions, physical sensations, and automatic behaviors rather than conscious recollection.

Inflammatory Response – The immune system's reaction to injury or infection. Chronic trauma can lead to persistent inflammation throughout the body, contributing to various health problems.

Learned Helplessness – A psychological phenomenon where repeated exposure to uncontrollable stressful situations leads to a sense of powerlessness and failure to escape even when escape becomes possible. Demonstrated through research by S.F. Maier and M.E. Seligman.

Leaden Paralysis – A symptom where individuals feel as if their arms and legs are made of lead and it's difficult to move them, often related to mitochondrial dysfunction in muscles.

Locus Coeruleus – A brain region that releases noradrenaline during stress, which can disrupt the brain's ability to manage instincts and impulses.

Mitochondria – Microscopic structures within cells that serve as cellular powerhouses, converting food and oxygen into usable energy (ATP). They play crucial roles in energy production, neurotransmitter synthesis, inflammation control, stress response, and gene expression. Chronic cortisol exposure from childhood trauma can damage mitochondria, leading to widespread mental and physical health problems.

Mitochondrial Biogenesis – The creation of new mitochondria, which can be stimulated through exercise, quality nutrition, restorative sleep, and stress management.

Mitochondrial Dysfunction – Impaired function of mitochondria, often resulting from chronic stress and trauma. Can manifest as chronic fatigue, cognitive problems, mood disorders, and various physical health issues.

Neuroplasticity - The brain's ability to reorganize and form new neural connections throughout life. This capacity for change provides hope for trauma recovery, as the brain can be "rewired" through appropriate interventions.

Neurotransmitters - Chemical messengers in the brain (such as serotonin, dopamine, and GABA) that regulate mood, motivation, and emotional states. Mitochondrial dysfunction from trauma can impair neurotransmitter production.

Noradrenaline (Norepinephrine) - A stress hormone and neurotransmitter that increases alertness and arousal. High levels can disrupt impulse control and decision-making.

Numbing - An emotional state where individuals feel detached from their emotions, unable to experience positive or negative feelings fully. Common in trauma survivors as a protective mechanism.

Parasympathetic Nervous System (PNS) - The part of the nervous system responsible for "rest and digest" functions. When activated, it promotes calm, connection, and healing—the opposite of the stress response.

Population Attributable Fraction - An epidemiological measure that calculates what percentage of disease or death in a population would be prevented if a specific risk factor were eliminated.

Post-Traumatic Stress Disorder (PTSD) - A mental health condition triggered by experiencing or witnessing a traumatic event, characterized by intrusive memories, avoidance behaviors, negative changes in thinking and mood, and alterations in arousal and reactivity.

Prefrontal Cortex - The brain region responsible for executive functions such as decision-making, impulse control, and emotional regulation. Trauma can impair the development and functioning of this critical area, leading to difficulties with concentration, problem-solving, and behavioral control.

Prevalence - In epidemiological terms, the total number of existing cases of a condition in a specific population at a given time, usually expressed as a percentage.

Resilience - The ability to adapt, bounce back, and grow in the face of adversity. Resilience can be developed through various interventions, supportive relationships, and by addressing trauma.

The Sacred Sixty - A term referring to the first 60 days of life, during which the quality of attachment and nurturing can profoundly influence a child's neurobiological development and future resilience. Research shows this period is more critical than previously understood, with neglect during this time potentially more damaging than later trauma.

SAM Axis (Sympathoadrenal Medullary Axis) - The part of the stress response system that triggers the immediate release of adrenaline from the adrenal glands.

Secondary Trauma (Vicarious Trauma) - The emotional and psychological impact experienced by individuals who are indirectly exposed to traumatic experiences of others, often affecting caregivers, therapists, siblings of traumatized children, and family members.

Somatic - Relating to the body and physical sensations. Somatic approaches to trauma therapy focus on the body's responses and stored trauma rather than primarily on thoughts and emotions.

State-Dependent Stress - When stress or reminders of past trauma trigger implicit or explicit memories along with the original emotions, sensations, and physical responses.

Stress Hormones - Hormones such as cortisol, adrenaline, and noradrenaline released during the stress response. Chronic elevation can cause widespread damage to body systems.

Sympathetic Nervous System (SNS) - The part of the nervous system that activates the fight-or-flight response during perceived threats, increasing heart rate, blood pressure, and stress hormone production.

Synaptogenesis - The formation of synapses (connections) between neurons in the brain. This process is particularly active in early childhood and can be disrupted by trauma.

Toxic Stress - Prolonged activation of the stress response system in the absence of protective relationships. Unlike normal stress, toxic stress can disrupt brain architecture, damage mitochondria, and affect other organ systems throughout life.

Trauma-Informed Care - An approach that recognizes and responds to the widespread impact of trauma, emphasizing safety, trustworthiness, collaboration, and empowerment in all interactions.

Triggers - Stimuli (sounds, smells, situations, etc.) that activate traumatic memories and stress responses, often causing a person to react as if the original trauma is happening again.

UACT (United Against Childhood Trauma) - The organization founded by the author dedicated to raising awareness, promoting healing, and preventing childhood trauma through collective action and advocacy.

Years of Potential Life Lost (YPLL) - An epidemiological measure that quantifies the impact of premature mortality by calculating the total number of years lost due to early deaths from a specific cause, providing insight into the societal burden of health conditions. Research shows individuals with six or more ACEs die an average of 20 years earlier than those without ACEs.

Recommended Reading

The Adverse Childhood Experiences Recovery Workbook

Glenn R. Schiraldi, PhD

Powerful new strategies to help heal the hidden wounds from childhood affecting your adult mental and physical health.

The Resilience Workbook

Glenn R. Schiraldi, PhD

Invaluable insights and essential skills to help you bounce back from setbacks and cultivate a growth mindset.

The Deepest Well

Dr. Nadine Harris Burke

This book explores the profound impact of childhood trauma on life-long health, weaving together compelling research, personal stories, and actionable insights to highlight the importance of understanding and addressing adverse childhood experiences.

The Body Keeps the Score

Dr. Bessel van der Kolk

This book covers the intricate relationship between trauma and the body, illustrating how adverse experiences affect both mental and physical health while offering innovative treatments to reclaim self-awareness and healing.

The Unexpected Gift of Trauma: The Path to Posttraumatic Growth
Dr. Edith Shiro

A groundbreaking approach to healing from trauma and experiencing posttraumatic growth from a leading psychologist, featuring a powerful, five-stage framework to help readers not just recover but thrive and transform.

What Happened to You? Conversations on Trauma, Resilience, and Healing
Bruce D. Perry, MD, PhD and Oprah Winfrey

Our earliest experiences shape our lives far down the road. This book provides powerful scientific and emotional insights into behavioral patterns that many of us struggle to understand.

Own Your Past, Change Your Future
Dr. John Delony

We are all carrying the weight of our trauma based on our stories—and those stories are like bricks in a backpack that keeps us from being happy and healthy. In his book, Dr. Delony provides a clear, five-step path to being well.

GRIT: The Power of Passion and Perseverance
Angela Duckworth

Learn that the secret to outstanding achievement is not talent but a unique blend of passion and persistence that Angela Duckworth calls "GRIT."

What My Bones Know: A Memoir of Healing from Complex Trauma
Stephanie Foo

A memoir of reckoning and healing from the investigation of the little-understood science behind complex PTSD and how it shaped the author's life.

Trauma Through a Child's Eyes
Peter A. Levine and Maggie Kline

An essential guide for recognizing, preventing, and healing childhood trauma from infancy through adolescence—what parents, educators, and health professionals can do.

The Drama of the Gifted Child
Alice Miller

Why are many of the most successful people plagued by feelings of emptiness and alienation? This wise and profound book has provided millions of readers with an answer—and has helped them to apply it to their own lives.

Spark: The Revolutionary New Science of Exercise and the Brain
Dr. John Ratey

This book embarks upon a fascinating and entertaining journey through the mind-body connection, presenting startling research to prove that exercise is truly our best defense against everything from depression to ADD to addiction to aggression to menopause to Alzheimer's.

Positive Discipline

Jane Nelson

Help for parents who lack parenting skills raise responsible, respectful children, balancing kindness and firmness, and treating them with dignity and respect.

Helpful Websites:

Center for Disease Control—CDC.gov

National Child Traumatic Stress Network—NCTSN.org

Early Childhood Mental Health Consultation—ECMHC.org

National Institute for Children's Health Quality—NICHQ.org

References

1. Murphy, S. L., et al. "Mortality in the United States, 2023." NCHS Data Brief, no. 521. CDC, 2024.

2. Kelly-Irving, M., et al. "Adverse Childhood Experiences and Premature All-Cause Mortality." European Journal of Epidemiology 28 (2013): 721–34.

3. Swedo, Elizabeth A., Sherry A. Sumner, Susan D. Hillis, et al. "Adverse Childhood Experiences and Health Conditions and Risk Behaviors Among High School Students—Youth Risk Behavior Survey, United States, 2023." MMWR Morbidity and Mortality Weekly Report 73, Suppl-4 (2024): 1–10.

4. Leza, L., et al. "Adverse Childhood Experiences (ACEs) and Substance Use Disorder (SUD): A Scoping Review." Drug and Alcohol Dependence 221 (2021): 108563.

5. Peterson, C., et al. "Lifetime Economic Burden of Intimate Partner Violence Among US Adults." American Journal of Preventive Medicine 55, no. 4 (2018): 433–44.

6. Wilson, R. F., et al. "Trends in Homicide Rates for US Children Aged 0 to 17 Years, 1999 to 2020." JAMA Pediatrics 177, no. 2 (2023): 187–97.

7. Bohm, David. Wholeness and the Implicate Order. London: Routledge & Kegan Paul, 1980.

8. Felitti, Vincent J., Robert F. Anda, Dale Nordenberg, David F. Williamson, Alison M. Spitz, Valerie Edwards, Mary P. Koss, and James S. Marks. "Relationship of Childhood Abuse and Household Dysfunction to Many of the Leading Causes of Death in Adults: The Adverse Childhood Experiences (ACE) Study." American Journal of Preventive Medicine 14, no. 4 (1998): 245–58.

9. Schiraldi, Glenn R. The Adverse Childhood Experiences Recovery Workbook. Oakland, CA: New Harbinger Publications, 2021.

10. Perry, Bruce D., and Maia Szalavitz. The Boy Who Was Raised as a Dog: And Other Stories from a Child Psychiatrist's Notebook—What Traumatized Children Can Teach Us About Loss, Love, and Healing. New York: Basic Books, 2006. Rev. ed., 2017.

11. Liedloff, Jean. The Continuum Concept: In Search of Happiness Lost. Cambridge, MA: Da Capo Press, 1975.

12. Greenspan, Stanley I., and Stuart G. Shanker. The First Idea: How Symbols, Language, and Intelligence Evolved from Our Primate Ancestors to Modern Humans. Cambridge, MA: Da Capo Press, 2004.

13. Cataudella, Stefania, et al. "From Pregnancy to 3 Months After Birth: The Beginning of Mother-Infant Relationship from a Maternal Perspective." Infant Mental Health Journal 40, no. 3

(July 2022): 266–87.

14. Hambrick, Erin P., Thomas W. Brawner, Bruce D. Perry, Kristie Brandt, Christine Hofmeister, and Jen O. Collins. "Beyond the ACE Score: Examining Relationships Between Timing of Developmental Adversity, Relational Health and Developmental Outcomes in Children." Archives of Psychiatric Nursing 33, no. 3 (2019): 238–47. https://doi.org/10.1016/j.apnu.2018.11.001.

15. Hughes, K., M. A. Bellis, K. A. Hardcastle, D. Sethi, A. Butchart, C. Mikton, L. Jones, and M. P. Dunne. "The Effect of Multiple Adverse Childhood Experiences on Health: A Systematic Review and Meta-Analysis." Lancet Public Health 2, no. 8 (August 2017): e356–e366. https://doi.org/10.1016/S2468-2667(17)30118-4.

16. Bruce, J., P. A. Fisher, K. C. Pears, and S. Levine. "Morning Cortisol Levels in Preschool-Aged Foster Children: Differential Effects of Maltreatment Type." Developmental Psychobiology 51, no. 1 (2009): 14–23. https://doi.org/10.1002/dev.20333.

17. van der Kolk, Bessel A. The Body Keeps the Score: Brain, Mind, and Body in the Healing of Trauma. New York: Viking, 2014.

18. Tottenham, N., T. A. Hare, B. T. Quinn, T. W. McCarry, M. Nurse, T. Gilhooly, A. Millner, A. Galvan, M. C. Davidson, I. M. Eigsti, K. M. Thomas, P. J. Freed, E. S. Booma, M. R. Gunnar, M. Altemus, J. Aronson, and B. J. Casey. "Prolonged Institutional Rearing Is Associated with Atypically Large Amygdala Volume and Difficulties in Emotion Regulation." Develop-

mental Science 13, no. 1 (2010): 46–61. https://doi.org/10.1 111/j.1467-7687.2009.00852.x.

19. Danese, Andrea, Carmine M. Pariante, Avshalom Caspi, Alan Taylor, and Richie Poulton. "Childhood Maltreatment Predicts Adult Inflammation in a Life-Course Study." *Proceedings of the National Academy of Sciences* 104, no. 4 (2007): 1319–24. https://doi.org/10.1073/pnas.0610362104.

20. Palmer, Christopher M. Brain Energy: A Revolutionary Breakthrough in Understanding Mental Health—and Improving Treatment for Anxiety, Depression, OCD, PTSD, and More. Dallas: BenBella Books, 2022.

21. Grummitt LR, Kreski NT, Kim SG, Platt J, Keyes KM, McLaughlin KA. Association of Childhood Adversity With Morbidity and Mortality in US Adults: A Systematic Review. JAMA Pediatrics. 2021;175(12):1269-1278. doi:10.1001/jama pediatrics.2021.2320

22. Merrick, Melissa T., Derek C. Ford, Katie A. Ports, et al. "Vital Signs: Estimated Proportion of Adult Health Problems Attributable to Adverse Childhood Experiences and Implications for Prevention—25 States, 2015–2017." MMWR Morbidity and Mortality Weekly Report 68 (2019): 999–1005.

23. Austin AE, et al. Adolescent Opioid Misuse Attributable to Adverse Childhood Experiences. Journal of Pediatrics. 2020;224:102-109. doi:10.1016/j.jpeds.2020.05.001

24. Dube, Shanta R., et al. "Childhood Abuse, Household Dysfunction and the Risk of Illicit Drug Use." Pediatrics 111, no.

3 (2003): 564–72.

25. U.S. Department of Health and Human Services, Administration for Children and Families, Children's Bureau. Child Maltreatment 2022. 2024. Available at: acf.hhs.gov/cb/data-research/child-maltreatment

26. Zheng L, et al. Association between adverse childhood experiences and mortality: A systematic review and meta-analysis. Psychiatry Research. 2025;343:116275. doi:10.1016/j.psychres.2024.116275

27. CDC Office on Smoking and Health. Tobacco-Related Mortality. 2024. Available at: cdc.gov/tobacco

28. Mokdad AH, Marks JS, Stroup DF, Gerberding JL. Actual Causes of Death in the United States, 2000. JAMA. 2004;291(10):1238-1245. doi:10.1001/jama.291.10.1238

29. CDC. Deaths from Excessive Alcohol Use — United States, 2016–2021. MMWR. 2024;73(8):154-161.

30. University of Minnesota. "Adverse Childhood Experiences and Opioid Crisis." 2023.

31. Lund, Ingunn Olea, et al. "Adverse Childhood Experiences and Substance Use Disorders in Adulthood: Young-HUNT Study." Addiction 118 (2023): 44–56.

32. American Counseling Association. "The Intersection of Childhood Trauma and Addiction." 2023.

33. "Adverse Childhood Experiences and Health Conditions

Among High School Students—YRBS 2023." MMWR Morbidity and Mortality Weekly Report 73, SS-4 (2024): 1–10.

34. Brown, David W., et al. "Adverse Childhood Experiences and Suicide Attempts in a National Sample." JAMA Psychiatry 67 (2019): 1135–42.

35. Extrapolated from mitochondrial dysfunction studies in trauma survivors.

36. Reavis, James A., et al. "Adverse Childhood Experiences and Adult Criminality." Permanente Journal 17, no. 2 (2013): 44–48.

37. Compassion Prison Project. "Childhood Trauma Statistics." 2024.

38. Turney, Kristin. "Adverse Childhood Experiences Among Children of Incarcerated Parents." Children and Youth Services Review 89 (2018): 218–25.

39. SAMHSA. "National Survey on Drug Use and Health." 2023.

40. Bellis, Mark A., Karen Hughes, Kat Ford, et al. "Life Course Health Consequences and Associated Annual Costs of Adverse Childhood Experiences Across Europe and North America: A Systematic Review and Meta-Analysis." Lancet Public Health 4 (2019): e517–e528.

41. Maier, Steven F., and Martin E. Seligman. "Learned Helplessness: Theory and Evidence." Journal of Experimental Psychology: General 105, no. 1 (1976): 3–46. See also Seligman, Martin E., Steven F. Maier, and James H. Geer. "Alleviation of Learned

Helplessness in the Dog." Journal of Abnormal Psychology 73, no. 3 (1968): 256–62; and Jackson, R. L., J. H. Alexander, and Steven F. Maier. "Learned Helplessness, Inactivity, and Associative Deficits: Effects of Inescapable Shock on Response Choice Escape Learning." Journal of Experimental Psychology: Animal Behavior Processes 6, no. 1 (1980): 1–20.

42. Maier, Steven F., and Martin E. Seligman. "Learned Helplessness: Theory and Evidence." Journal of Experimental Psychology: General 105, no. 1 (1976): 3–46. See also Seligman, Martin E., Steven F. Maier, and James H. Geer. "Alleviation of Learned Helplessness in the Dog." Journal of Abnormal Psychology 73, no. 3 (1968): 256–62; and Jackson, R. L., J. H. Alexander, and Steven F. Maier. "Learned Helplessness, Inactivity, and Associative Deficits: Effects of Inescapable Shock on Response Choice Escape Learning." Journal of Experimental Psychology: Animal Behavior Processes 6, no. 1 (1980): 1–20.

43. Trickett, Penelope K., Jennie G. Noll, and Frank W. Putnam. "The Impact of Sexual Abuse on Female Development: Lessons from a Multigenerational, Longitudinal Research Study." Development and Psychopathology 23 (2011): 453–76.

44. Kessler, Ronald C., et al. "The Epidemiology of Major Depressive Disorders in the General Population: Results from the National Comorbidity Survey Replication."

45. Caspi, Avshalom, Terrie E. Moffitt, HonaLee Harrington, Barry J. Milne, Richie Poulton, and Alan Taylor. "Children's Behavioral Styles at Age 3 Are Linked to Their Adult Personality Traits at Age 26." Journal of Personality 71, no. 4 (2003):

495–513. https://doi.org/10.1111/1467-6494.7104001.

46. Green, Jennifer G., Katie A. McLaughlin, Patricia A. Berglund, Michael J. Gruber, Nancy A. Sampson, Alan M. Zaslavsky, Ronald C. Kessler, with Margarita Alegria, E. Jane Costello, Michael Gruber, Nancy Sampson, Ronald C. Kessler, Kathleen R. Merikangas, Beth Pennell, Alan M. Zaslavsky, Shelli Avenevoli, E. Jane Costello, Doreen Koretz, Ronald C. Kessler, … Avshalom Caspi, and Terrie E. Moffitt. "Childhood Adversities and Adult Psychiatric Disorders in the National Comorbidity Survey Replication I: Associations with First Onset of DSM-IV Disorders." Archives of General Psychiatry 67, no. 2 (2010): 113–23. https://doi.org/10.1001/archgenpsychiatry.2009.186.

47. Strassnig, Martin, Roman Kotov, Danielle Cornaccio, Laura Fochtmann, Philip D. Harvey, and Evelyn J. Bromet. "Twenty-Year Progression of Body Mass Index in a County-Wide Cohort of People with Schizophrenia and Bipolar Disorder Identified at Their First Episode of Psychosis." Bipolar Disorders 19, no. 5 (2017): 336–43. https://doi.org/10.1111/bdi.12505.

48. Afzal, M., N. Siddiqi, B. Ahmad, N. Afsheen, F. Aslam, A. Ali, R. Ayesha, M. Bryant, R. Holt, H. Khalid, K. Ishaq, K. N. Koly, S. Rajan, J. Saba, N. Tirbhowan, and G. A. Zavala. "Prevalence of Overweight and Obesity in People with Severe Mental Illness: Systematic Review and Meta-Analysis." Frontiers in Endocrinology 12 (2021): 769309. https://doi.org/10.3389/fendo.2021.769309.

49. Brown, David W., Robert F. Anda, Henning Tiemeier, Vincent J. Felitti, Valerie J. Edwards, Janet B. Croft, and Wayne H. Giles. "Adverse Childhood Experiences and the Risk of Premature Death." American Journal of Preventive Medicine 37, no. 5 (2009): 389–96.

50. Picard, Martin, and Bruce S. McEwen. "Psychological Stress and Mitochondria: A Systematic Review." Psychosomatic Medicine 80, no. 2 (2018): 141–53.

51. Herculano-Houzel, Suzana. "The Remarkable, Yet Not Extraordinary, Human Brain as a Scaled-Up Primate Brain and Its Associated Cost." Proceedings of the National Academy of Sciences 109, Suppl. 1 (2012): 10661–68.

52. Kann, Oliver, and Richard Kovács. "Mitochondria and Neuronal Activity." American Journal of Physiology-Cell Physiology 292, no. 2 (2007): C641–57.

53. Hunter, Richard G., Kristina Gagnidze, Bruce S. McEwen, and Donald W. Pfaff. "Stress and the Dynamic Genome: Steroids, Epigenetics, and the Transposome." Proceedings of the National Academy of Sciences 112, no. 22 (2015): 6828–33.

54. Bowers, Meaghan E., and Rachel Yehuda. "Intergenerational Transmission of Stress in Humans." Neuropsychopharmacology 41, no. 1 (2016): 232–44.

55. Nicolson, Garth L. "Mitochondrial Dysfunction and Chronic Disease: Treatment with Natural Supplements." Integrative Medicine 13, no. 4 (2014): 35–43.

56. Lieberman, Alicia F., Patricia Van Horn, and Chandra Ghosh Ippen. "Toward Evidence-Based Treatment: Child-Parent Psychotherapy with Preschoolers Exposed to Marital Violence." Journal of the American Academy of Child & Adolescent Psychiatry 44, no. 12 (2005): 1241–48. https://doi.org/10.1097/01.chi.0000181047.59702.58.

57. Brown, David W., Robert A. Anda, Vincent J. Felitti, et al. "Adverse Childhood Experiences Are Associated with the Risk of Lung Cancer: A Prospective Cohort Study." BMC Public Health 10 (2010): 20–32. Accessed July 24, 2013. http://www.biomedcentral.com/1471-2458/10/20.

58. Danese, Andrea, and Bruce S. McEwen. "Adverse Childhood Experiences, Allostasis, Allostatic Load, and Age-Related Disease." Physiology & Behavior 106, no. 1 (2012): 29–39. https://doi.org/10.1016/j.physbeh.2011.08.019.

59. Baumeister, David, Raees Akhtar, Simone Ciufolini, Carmine M. Pariante, and Valeria Mondelli. "Childhood Trauma and Adulthood Inflammation: A Meta-Analysis of Peripheral C-Reactive Protein, Interleukin-6 and Tumour Necrosis Factor-α." Molecular Psychiatry 21, no. 5 (2016): 642–49. https://doi.org/10.1038/mp.2015.67.

60. Hostinar, Camelia E., Robin Nusslock, and Gregory E. Miller. "Future Directions in the Study of Early-Life Stress and Physical and Emotional Health: Implications of the Neuroimmune Network Hypothesis." Journal of Clinical Child & Adolescent Psychology 47, no. 1 (2018): 142–56. https://doi.org/10.1080/15374416.2016.1266647.

61. Ports, Katie A., Donatus M. Holman, Angie S. Guinn, Satvinder Pampati, Kayla E. Dyer, Melissa T. Merrick, Natalie B. Lunsford, and Marilyn Metzler. "Adverse Childhood Experiences and the Presence of Cancer Risk Factors in Adulthood: A Scoping Review of the Literature From 2005 to 2015." Journal of Pediatric Nursing 44 (2018): 81–96. https://doi.org/10.1016/j.pedn.2018.10.009.

62. Alimujiang, Aliya, Andrea Wiensch, Jonathan Boss, et al. "Association Between Life Purpose and Mortality Among US Adults Older Than 50 Years." JAMA Network Open 2, no. 5 (2019): e194270. https://doi.org/10.1001/jamanetworkopen.2019.4270.

63. Maté, Gabor. In the Realm of Hungry Ghosts: Close Encounters with Addiction. Berkeley, CA: North Atlantic Books, 2010.

64. U.S. Department of Justice, Office of Justice Programs. "Child's Table: Indicators of School Crime and Safety." Bureau of Justice Statistics Special Report. Washington, DC: U.S. Government Printing Office, 2006.

65. Harper, Cynthia, and Sara S. McLanahan. "Father Absence and Youth Incarceration." Journal of Research on Adolescence 14, no. 3 (2004): 369–97. https://doi.org/10.1111/j.1532-7795.2004.00079.x.

66. Wolff, Nancy, and Jing Shi. "Childhood and Adult Trauma Experiences of Incarcerated Persons and Their Relationship to Adult Behavioral Health Problems and Treatment." International Journal of Environmental Research and Public Health 9, no. 5 (2012): 1908–26. https://doi.org/10.3390/ijerph9051908.

67. Baglivio, Michael T., Nathan Epps, Kimberly Swartz, Mona S. Huq, Amy Sheer, and Nancy S. Hardt. "The Prevalence of Adverse Childhood Experiences (ACEs) in the Lives of Juvenile Offenders." Journal of Juvenile Justice 3, no. 2 (2014): 1–23.

68. Peterson, Cora, Curtis Florence, and Joanne Klevens. "The Economic Burden of Child Maltreatment in the United States, 2015." Child Abuse & Neglect 86 (2018): 178–83. https://doi .org/10.1016/j.chiabu.2018.09.018.

69. Merrick, Melissa T., Derek C. Ford, Katie A. Ports, et al. "Vital Signs: Estimated Proportion of Adult Health Problems Attrib-utable to Adverse Childhood Experiences and Implications for Prevention—25 States, 2015–2017." MMWR Morbidity and Mortality Weekly Report 68 (2019): 999–1005.

70. American Cancer Society. Cancer Facts & Figures 2023. At-lanta: American Cancer Society, 2023.

71. Peterson, Cora, Curtis Florence, and Joanne Klevens. "The Economic Burden of Health Conditions Associated with Ad-verse Childhood Experiences Among US Adults." JAMA Net-work Open 6, no. 1 (2023): e2251661.

72. Danese, Andrea, Terrie E. Moffitt, HonaLee Harrington, et al. "The Origins of Cognitive Deficits in Victimized Chil-dren: Implications for Neuroscientists and Clinicians." Ameri-can Journal of Psychiatry 174 (2017): 349–61.

73. Peterson, Cora, Curtis Florence, and Joanne Klevens. "Eco-nomic Burden of Health Conditions Associated with Adverse Childhood Experiences—Tennessee, 2019." American Journal

of Preventive Medicine 55, no. 6 (2018): 823–32.

74. Based on CDC prevalence data: 63.9% of adults report at least one ACE, with 17.3% reporting four or more ACEs.

75. Chartier, Mariette J., John R. Walker, and Bernard Naimark. "Separate and Cumulative Effects of Adverse Childhood Experiences in Predicting Adult Health and Health Care Utilization." Child Abuse & Neglect 34 (2010): 454–64.

76. Anda, Robert F., Vincent J. Felitti, J. Douglas Bremner, et al. "The Enduring Effects of Abuse and Related Adverse Experiences in Childhood." European Archives of Psychiatry and Clinical Neuroscience 256 (2006): 174–86.

77. Felitti, Vincent J., Robert F. Anda, Dale Nordenberg, et al. "Relationship of Childhood Abuse and Household Dysfunction to Many of the Leading Causes of Death in Adults." American Journal of Preventive Medicine 14 (1998): 245–58.

78. Brown, David W., Robert F. Anda, Henning Tiemeier, et al. "Adverse Childhood Experiences and the Risk of Premature Mortality." American Journal of Preventive Medicine 37 (2009): 389–96.

79. Raja, Saira, Mahvish Hasnain, Michelle Hoersch, et al. "Trauma Informed Care in Medicine: Current Knowledge and Future Research Directions." Family & Community Health 38 (2015): 216–26.

80. "Philadelphia ACE Survey." ACES Philadelphia, 2012. https://www.philadelphiaaces.org/philadelphia-ace-survey.

81. Steuwe, Carolin, et al. "Effect of Direct Eye Contact in PTSD Related to Interpersonal Trauma: An MRI Study of Activation of an Innate Alarm System." Social Cognitive and Affective Neuroscience 9, no. 1 (January 2014): 88–97.

82. National Center for Health Statistics. "Years of Potential Life Lost." Centers for Disease Control and Prevention, 2023.

83. Menard, M. "The Economic Burden of Adverse Childhood Experiences: A Comprehensive Analysis of Healthcare and Societal Costs." Author's calculations based on CDC BRFSS data, trauma prevalence rates, and years of life lost methodology. UACT Research Series, 2025.

84. McLanahan, Sara, Laura Tach, and Daniel Schneider. "The Causal Effects of Father Absence." Annual Review of Sociology 39 (2013): 399–427. https://doi.org/10.1146/annurev-soc-071312-145704.

85. Amato, Paul R., and Bruce Keith. "Parental Divorce and the Well-Being of Children: A Meta-Analysis." Psychological Bulletin 110, no. 1 (1991): 26–46. https://doi.org/10.1037/0033-2909.110.1.26.

86. National Fatherhood Initiative. Father Facts. 8th ed. Germantown, MD: National Fatherhood Initiative, 2020.

87. World Health Organization. Global Status Report on Preventing Violence Against Children. Geneva: World Health Organization, 2020.

88. Hillis, Susan, James Mercy, Adaugo Amobi, and Howard Kress.

"Global Prevalence of Past-Year Violence Against Children: A Systematic Review and Minimum Estimates." Pediatrics 137, no. 3 (2016): e20154079. https://doi.org/10.1542/peds.2015-4079.

89. U.S. Department of Health and Human Services, Administration for Children and Families. (2024). The AFCARS Report: Preliminary FY 2023 Estimates.

90. Christian Alliance for Orphans (CAFO). (2025). US Foster Care Statistics 2025: Data & Trends. Retrieved from cafo.org/foster-care-statistics/

91. Leathers, S. J., Spielfogel, J. E., Geiger, J., Barnett, J., & Vande Voort, B. L. (2019). Placement disruption in foster care: Children's behavior, foster parent support, and parenting experiences. Child Abuse & Neglect, 91, 59–68. See also: James, S. (2004). Why do foster care placements disrupt? An investigation of reasons for placement change in foster care. Social Service Review, 78(4), 601–627.

92. National Conference of State Legislatures (NCSL). (2022). Foster Parent Retention. Retrieved from ncsl.org. See also: Wulczyn, F., Orlebeke, B., & Haight, J. (2018). The Dynamics of Foster Home Recruitment and Retention. Chapin Hall Center for State Child Welfare Data, University of Chicago.

93. Sanctuary Foster Care Services. (2024). Foster Care Statistics: Placement Disruption Data. Retrieved from sanctuaryfostercare.org/stats

94. Oosterman, M., Schuengel, C., Slot, N. W., Bullens, R. A., &

Doreleijers, T. A. (2007). Disruptions in foster care: A review and meta-analysis. Children and Youth Services Review, 29(1), 53–76.

95. McEwen, B. S. (1998). Stress, adaptation, and disease: Allostasis and allostatic load. Annals of the New York Academy of Sciences, 840(1), 33–44.

96. Shonkoff, J. P., Garner, A. S., et al. (2012). The lifelong effects of early childhood adversity and toxic stress. Pediatrics, 129(1), e232–e246.

97. Lancy, David F. The Anthropology of Childhood: Cherubs, Chattel, Changelings. Cambridge: Cambridge University Press, 2015.

98. Yehuda, Rachel, and Amy Lehrner. "Intergenerational Transmission of Trauma Effects: Putative Role of Epigenetic Mechanisms." World Psychiatry 17, no. 3 (2018): 243–57.

99. Farmer, Paul. "An Anthropology of Structural Violence." Current Anthropology 45, no. 3 (2004): 305–25.

100. Worthman, Carol M., and Catherine Panter-Brick. "Homeless Street Children in Nepal: Use of Allostatic Load to Assess the Burden of Childhood Adversity." Development and Psychopathology 20, no. 1 (2008): 233–55.

101. Kleinman, Arthur, Veena Das, and Margaret Lock, eds. Social Suffering. Berkeley: University of California Press, 1997.

102. Collins, Patricia Hill. Intersectionality as Critical Social Theory. Durham, NC: Duke University Press, 2019.

103. Corsaro, William A. The Sociology of Childhood. 5th ed. Thousand Oaks, CA: SAGE Publications, 2017.

104. Putnam, Robert D. Bowling Alone: The Collapse and Revival of American Community. New York: Simon & Schuster, 2000.

105. Gerbner, George, Larry Gross, Michael Morgan, Nancy Signorielli, and James Shanahan. "Growing Up with Television: Cultivation Processes." In Media Effects: Advances in Theory and Research, edited by Jennings Bryant and Dolf Zillmann, 43–67. Mahwah, NJ: Lawrence Erlbaum Associates, 2002.

106. Elder, Glen H., Jr., Monica Kirkpatrick Johnson, and Robert Crosnoe. "The Emergence and Development of Life Course Theory." In Handbook of the Life Course, edited by Jeylan T. Mortimer and Michael J. Shanahan, 3–19. New York: Springer, 2003.

107. Judd, Lewis L., Hagop S. Akiskal, Janet D. Maser, et al. "A Prospective 12-Year Study of Subsyndromal and Syndromal Depressive Symptoms in Unipolar Major Depressive Disorders." Archives of General Psychiatry 55, no. 8 (1998): 694–700. https://doi.org/10.1001/archpsyc.55.8.694.

108. Dr. Tom Insel, the former director of the National Institute of Mental Health.

109. Burke Harris, Nadine. The Deepest Well: Healing the Long-Term Effects of Childhood Adversity. Boston: Houghton Mifflin Harcourt, 2018.

110. Humington, A., and Neuromastery Lab. The Neuroscience of

Gratitude: Why Self-Help Has It All Wrong: Rewire Your Brain With A Science-Backed Gratitude Practice in 5 Minutes A Day. NeuroMastery Lab Collection. Independently published, 2023.

111. Schiraldi, Glenn R. The Resilience Workbook: Essential Skills to Recover from Stress, Trauma, and Adversity. Oakland, CA: New Harbinger Publications, 2017.

112. Harvey, Allison G., and Fiona B. Taylor. "Sleep and Posttraumatic Stress Disorder: A Systematic Review and Meta-Analysis." Current Psychiatry Reports 12, no. 6 (2010): 467–75. https://doi.org/10.1007/s11920-010-0150-6.

113. Schore, Allan N. The Science of the Art of Psychotherapy. New York: W. W. Norton & Company, 2012.

114. Lewis, Thomas, Fari Amini, and Richard Lannon. A General Theory of Love. New York: Random House, 2000.

115. Lewis, Thomas, Fari Amini, and Richard Lannon. A General Theory of Love. New York: Random House, 2000.

116. Ratey, John J. Spark: The Revolutionary New Science of Exercise and the Brain. New York: Little, Brown and Company, 2008.

117. Neufeld, Gordon, and Gabor Maté. Hold On to Your Kids: Why Parents Need to Matter More Than Peers. New York: Ballantine Books, 2013.

118. Allegretto, Sylvia A., and Lawrence Mishel. "Teacher Pay Penalty Dips but Persists in 2019: Public School Teachers Earn

About 19.2% Less Than Similar Workers." Economic Policy Institute, September 17, 2020. https://www.epi.org/publication/teacher-pay-penalty-dips-but-persists-in-2019-public-school-teachers-earn-about-19-2-less-than-similar-workers/.

119. Doty, James R. Into the Magic Shop: A Neurosurgeon's Quest to Discover the Mysteries of the Brain and the Secrets of the Heart. New York: Avery, 2016.

120. Perry, Bruce D., and Ronnie Pollard. "Homeostasis, Stress, Trauma, and Adaptation: A Neurodevelopmental View of Childhood Trauma." Child and Adolescent Psychiatric Clinics of North America 7, no. 1 (1998): 33–51.

121. Davidson, Richard J., and Antoine Lutz. "Buddha's Brain: Neuroplasticity and Meditation." IEEE Signal Processing Magazine 25, no. 1 (2008): 176–74. https://doi.org/10.1109/MSP.2008.4431873.

About the Author

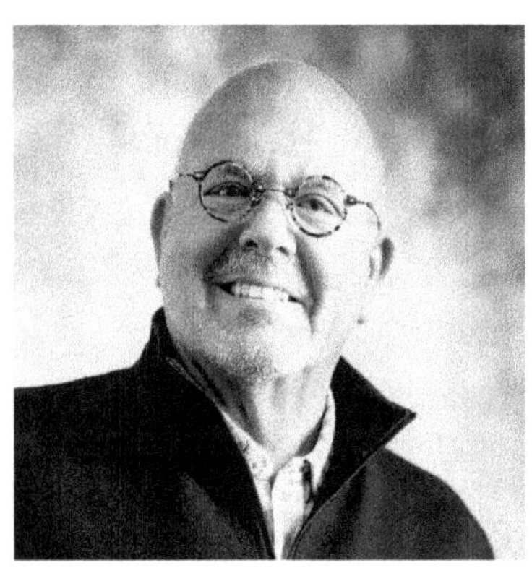

Michael Menard's journey from trauma survivor to the man who exposed the United States' leading cause of death represents one of the most important discoveries in modern public health.

Born into a family of 14 children in Kankakee, Illinois, Menard learned early that survival required both resilience and innovation. Despite growing up in a 900-square-foot home marked by poverty and dysfunction, he channeled his experiences into extraordinary achievement.

His engineering mind revolutionized industries. Over three decades in corporate leadership, Menard earned 14 patents that transformed global manufacturing, rising to worldwide Vice President of Engineering at Johnson & Johnson. His innovations touched millions of lives daily, proving his ability to solve complex problems at massive scale.

But his greatest discovery came much later. While writing his memoir *The Kite That Couldn't Fly* at age 72, Menard realized that what his family endured wasn't simply a "tough childhood"—it was complex trauma with devastating consequences that rippled through generations. Two brothers lost to addiction, multiple family members stalked by depression—each bearing invisible wounds that never healed.

Menard's engineer mind couldn't ignore the patterns. What began as personal revelation became intensive data analysis, ultimately revealing the shocking truth: severe childhood trauma is killing 1,401 Americans daily, a death toll that surpasses accidents, strokes, and diabetes combined.

The discovery that 89% of teen suicide attempts, 85-100% of addiction cases, and 90% of incarcerated individuals trace back to childhood trauma revealed the scope of this hidden epidemic. At a cost of $14 trillion annually—exceeding our defense budget—America faces its greatest public health crisis in history.

Rather than accept this devastating reality, Menard chose to expose and change it. He founded UACT (United Against Childhood Trauma) with an audacious goal: ending the deadliest force in the United States. His comprehensive plan includes awareness, healing, and prevention strategies designed to save those 1,401 daily lives.

Today, Menard brings the same systematic thinking that revolutionized industries to humanity's greatest challenge. His work has gained support from leading trauma experts, including Dr. Glenn Schiraldi, who calls childhood trauma "the largest threat to the well-being of humanity known today."

Menard lives in Tennessee with his wife, Emilie, whose background in early childhood development complements his mission. Together, they represent the powerful combination of lived experience, data analysis, and unwavering determination required to end America's hidden killer.

Explore more books by

Michael J Menard

A Fish in Your Ear
Corporate Transformation
The Kite That Couldn't Fly
Greater Than Gravity
Whispers of Hope
Bleeding in the Pews
Bleeding in the Boardroom

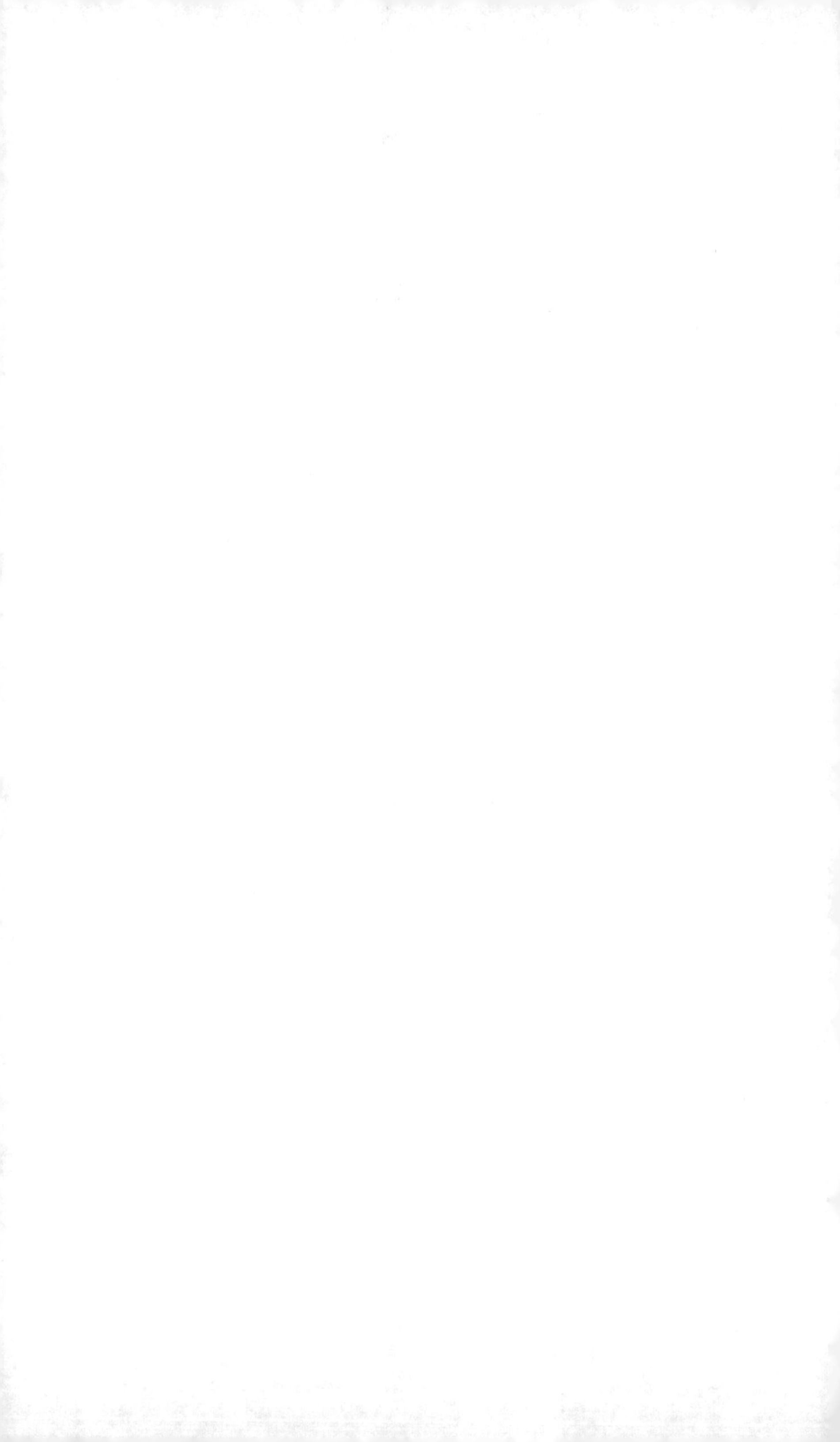